The
Sports
Injury
Handbook

Contents

Introduction

THE SPORTS INJURY HANDBOOK is the distillation of sixty years of clinical practice and medical experience by Dr. Hans Kraus, a truly extraordinary physician hailed by *The New York Times* as the "originator of sports medicine in the U.S."

As both physician and sportsman, Dr. Kraus knew what it took to guard against injury, to recover from injury—accidents do happen, as witness a sixty-foot fall he suffered climbing a cliff in the Shawangunk Mountains of New York—and to return to full activity. A former gymnast, fencer, and amateur boxer, he was a pioneer rock climber and mountaineer of international reputation with first ascents in the Alps, the Tetons and the Wind River Range in Wyoming, the Cascades in Washington, and the Bugaboos in British Columbia. Invited to join the first two American expeditions to Mount Everest, he reluctantly had to decline because of prior commitments—once because he was treating President Kennedy's back.

Hans was also an ardent cross-country skier—his wife, the former Madi Springer-Miller, was on the 1958 United States ski team—and he was elected to the Ski Hall of Fame for his medical contributions to that sport. Indeed, when skier Billy Kidd appeared on the cover of *Life* in 1970 after winning the first U.S. gold medal in the FIS World Championships, he presented an autographed copy of the cover to Hans with the inscription, "Thanks for putting me here." A skier, rock climber, and mountaineer until well into his seventies, Hans lived to ninety, and this book, his final testament, must serve as the bible for anyone involved in sports—amateur or pro, trainer or coach.

I say this as a longtime writer for *Sports Illustrated*, a very thankful patient, and as the editor of this book. I first met Hans in 1955 when I wrote an article for the magazine that reported on the study he did on the lack of physical fitness of American youngsters compared to their counterparts in Switzerland, Austria, and Italy. Hans presented the findings at the White House, and they caused Dwight Eisenhower to establish what became the President's Council on Physical Fitness and Sports. In 1980, the Council gave Hans its Distinguished Service Award.

In 1960, I injured my back. My first thought was to see Dr. Kraus, but he was climbing in British Columbia. So I saw an orthopedic surgeon who put me in traction in Manhattan's Columbia-Presbyterian Hospital for a week. During the next year and a half, I suffered increasingly frequent episodes of excruciating pain in both my back and left leg. Just turning a doorknob could send me to bed for a week, even though I was now wearing a back brace that I had to strap on each morning. Once when I suddenly fell to the kitchen floor in pain and was unable to rise, my wife had to get the local volunteer fire department to carry me upstairs to bed. I honestly thought I was going to be crippled for life.

The orthopedic surgeon thought that I needed disc surgery, but he wisely said—and this was unusual for an orthopod—that I should see Dr. Kraus for a second opinion. Hans looked at the X rays, examined me, and said that surgery was unnecessary. Instead of a disc problem, actually a rare disorder, he said that I had triggerpoints in a torn muscle, and after he eliminated them I would undergo exercise therapy. Meanwhile, I was to stop wearing the back brace because it was only worsening my condition. After that initial consultation, I saw Hans at his office twice a week to undergo treatment, and in several months I was a new man.

Unlike the majority of physicians who advocate rest, ice compression, and elevation, Hans used movement, ethyl chloride, and, when needed, elevation, to recover from injury. As he notes on page 73 in this book, "Rest does not promote healing, whereas movement does." He discovered that in the early 1930s while a fracture surgeon at the University of Vienna Hospital. There, he demonstrated that the patients who performed prescribed exercises made the best recoveries from fractures, even if they had suffered more severe fractures than patients who did not exercise at all.

Unfortunately, many physicians are not aware of the existence of triggerpoints, much less how they should be treated and eliminated, even though they can trigger disabling muscle pain. Tennis elbow is an example cited in this book. So is so-called "tendonitis," which puts pitchers, quarterbacks, and other athletes on the sidelines, the disabled list, or the bone pile of castoffs. Through the course of my career at *Sports Illustrated*, I saw any number of athletes who never reached their potential or had their careers cut short by injury. I often thought that some of them, perhaps most of them, were crippled by triggerpoints that doctors had failed to recognize, treat, and eliminate. Even today, I continue to think that if I had the money to buy a losing major league baseball club, or even a new franchise, I could quickly turn it into a winner by having Hans's associate, Dr. Norman Marcus, head of the New York Pain Treatment Program, recondition those cast aside because of supposedly permanent injury.

This is no daydream. In his book, *October 1964*, David Halberstam deals with the season in which the Cardinals wound up beating the Yankees in the World Series. On page 208, he writes that in 1963, Bill White, the Cards' first baseman, had hit 27 home runs, knocked in 109 runs, and batted .304, but in 1964 he was having an awful season. Afflicted with a shoulder injury, White blamed himself for the team's poor performance. Halberstam goes on to note that I knew Bill, and so I suggested that he see Dr. Kraus when the Cardinals came to New York to play the Mets.

Halberstam writes, "Kraus was famous, having helped treat John Kennedy for his chronic back problems. White went to see him, and Dr. Kraus immediately gave him a shot [a triggerpoint injection]. Unlike the team doctor, who had targeted an area in front of the shoulder, Dr. Kraus went after a spot in the back and

White felt immediate relief. A few days later, in a doubleheader in Pittsburgh, White celebrated by getting six hits, including two home runs, and knocking in five runs. The Cardinals swept the series. It was the kind of day a power hitter should have and which he had not had all year. A critical piece had been restored to the Cardinal lineup."

Disabling pain is often baffling to both patient and physician, but as Hans makes clear in this book on pages eight through thirteen, there are only four kinds of muscle pain: pain from triggerpoints, pain from muscle spasm, pain from muscle tension, and pain from muscle deficiency. Once the cause of the pain is identified, appropriate treatment can start, and recovery can be surprisingly rapid. A brief example: one Saturday when I was in my forties, I pulled a leg muscle playing touch football. On Monday morning, I hobbled into Hans's office in Manhattan, and ten days later I was running again. At the same time, a well-known NFL running back in his twenties suffered a similar pull, and he was out for most of the season.

Hans also treated every member of my family. When a surgeon said that my older son Peter, then fourteen, had Osgood Schlatter's disease and needed an operation for his knees, I took him to Hans for his evaluation. He said that an operation was absolutely unnecessary, and he had Peter go to a physical therapist at a hospital near us to do exercises that he prescribed. Peter turned out fine, but God knows what would have happened if he had undergone surgery.

When my daughter Stephanie was hospitalized locally with a painful lower back after she fell down a flight of stairs at home, the attending physician said that she would be immobilized for a month and unable to return to work for at least three months after that. Stephanie was in the hospital three days when I asked Hans, who was returning to the city from his weekend house, if he could stop by the hospital on his way back to see her. He did, and I watched as he had her do a few simple movements so he could check her condition. Suddenly the attending physician appeared in the room, and, stupidly, even arrogantly, he ordered

Hans to stop. I started to tell him who Dr. Kraus was, but he cut me off. Hans looked at me and said, "Sign Stephanie out of the hospital." I did. Back home, he had her do more movements, and a half hour later she walked downstairs. After three days of doing prescribed exercises, she returned to work.

Most recently my youngest, Alex, tore his right shoulder capsule loose while working as a float guide on the Snake River in Wyoming. An orthopedic surgeon put his arm in a sling, told him to rest, and then a week later said that Alex would need an operation. Alex flew east to get Dr. Kraus's opinion. When he arrived home, unbeknownst to me he went up to his room with a copy of the first edition of this book, removed the sling and began doing the shoulder exercises described here on pages 85 to 89. An hour later, Alex bounced downstairs and said, with a big grin, "Look at this, Dad," and began moving his shoulder up and down. Two days later on Monday, he saw Hans who told him to continue the exercises for four months and supplement them with weight training to regain strength before returning to work.

But kids are impatient. Alex flew back to Wyoming and on his own doubled up on the exercises and weight training. In two weeks he was back guiding on the Snake with almost full strength in his shoulder. "You crazy kid!" I shouted after he called to tell me what he had done. "You should have waited four weeks!" In any event, Alex was okay. Had he undergone the surgery the orthopod advised, he would have been sidelined and out of work for at least six months and possibly a year.

When Hans Kraus turned eighty-six, more than a hundred mountaineers and rock climbers from Maine to California gathered to honor him at a dinner at the Mohonk Mountain House in the Shawangunks. As James McCarthy, the toastmaster and a past president of the American Alpine Club, told *The New Yorker*, which ran an account of the dinner, "There's never been a turnout like this. Hans is multidimensional, a man for all seasons. He's a pioneer climber, a great innovative physician, and, of course, a former student of [James] Joyce's." To which Jon Ross, operator of a climbing school and guide service, added, "Hans is an extraordinary man who has done extraordinary things, but the incredible thing is that in no way does he perceive himself as someone special. And that just underlines his larger-than-life charisma for me."

Born in 1905 in Trieste, on the Adriatic Sea, where his father was in the shipping business, Hans was four when he clambered up his first hill, and at age eleven he climbed to the summit of his first high mountain, the 9,500-foot Vreneliasgartli in the Glarus Alps. Hans's father and mother wanted to learn English, so they hired a young Irish expatriate named James Joyce to give them private lessons at home.

Trieste was then under Austrian rule, and when Italy entered the First World War in 1915, the Kraus and Joyce families were evacuated to Zurich in neutral Switzerland. "In Zurich I went to the Joyces' apartment for language lessons once or twice a week," Hans recalled, "and there I met his wife, his daughter, Lucia, and his son, Giorgio. I remember that Mrs. Joyce would come in with a little cup of chamomile tea, and Joyce would soak a poultice in it and bathe his eyes. My parents and I knew that Joyce was a writer; I have copies of *Chamber Music* and *Dubliners* that he presented to them. He was not then the James Joyce that the world knows now, but I was greatly impressed by him. He was a very friendly and very charming man, who treated me like a grown-up, and not like a child, and he taught me not only English but Italian."

When the war ended, the Kraus family moved to Vienna, and by age sixteen Hans was climbing and leading others wherever he could in the Alps. One climb was not without tragedy. In a 1981 profile in *SI* by William Oscar Johnson, Hans recounted, "I knew nothing, and we had no equipment worthy of the name, and yet, for some reason, I didn't get killed doing it. I took a friend of mine up a twelve-thousand-foot mountain one day. We were putting up a first ascent on the face, and before the first ridge my friend fell. We had no pitons. We had no equipment. It was an unpardonable thing. I tried to hold the rope to keep him from falling. I gripped the rope as tight as I could, but, of course,

I could not stop him. The rope ripped and burned through my hands as he fell. My palms and fingers were denuded of their skin. They were stripped to the fascia. In some places the tendons showed."

His friend fell 2,000 feet, and Hans climbed down to him. "He was still warm, but there was no heartbeat. He had been killed. It was the first time that I had seen a dead person, and it changed me forever. I could do nothing for him. I continued on down toward the hut where other friends would be. It was a terrible trip. I fell into a crevasse, and I saved myself from dropping deep into the glacier only because I spread my arms to bridge the chasm.

"My hands were in terrible shape, bleeding heavily, and growing stiffer. The local doctor said I should be very happy to be alive, that I was incredibly lucky, but he also said that I would never be able to move my fingers again. He predicted that I would be equipped with stiffened claws because of what the rope had done to my hands. He bound them in bandages and said that was all that could be done."

Inadvertently, the tragedy gave Hans his first lesson in the value of movement in recovering from injury. "I began to soak my hands in hot water twice a day—each time I changed the bandages. As I soaked them, I moved the fingers. Slowly at first, painfully, they moved. But they did move. I kept it up. By some instinct, the idea of movement instead of immobilization worked for me. My hands were never quite perfect again, but I could move my fingers very well and I became adept at surgery. And, of course, I have climbed all my life, which requires strong and nimble fingers."

Hans's father wanted him to go into shipping, but Hans wanted to go to medical school. His father made him attend a commercial gymnasium, the equivalent of a business high school, instead of the classical gymnasium that prepared students for college, with college followed by medical school. Upon graduation from the commercial gymnasium, Hans worked during the day and went to night school for ten months. He then took eighteen examinations, not for college, but for direct admission to the University of Vienna Medical School, and got A's in all of them. His father finally relented.

After graduation, Hans was a fracture surgeon in the university hospital, and using ethyl chloride spray—a local anesthetic that temporarily eliminates muscle pain from sprains and strains to allow movement of the injured part—he devised exercise programs that enabled patients to recover quickly from injury. In 1932, when only twenty-seven and already serving as physician to several Austrian Olympic teams, he gave a paper on the use of the spray before the Academy of Physicians in Vienna. "I was just a young kid," he recalled. "They could have laughed me out of town, but they were very understanding." A correspondent for the *Journal of the American Medical Association* was very impressed by Hans's presentation, and he sent an abstract to the *Journal*, which published it. As a result, in 1934, surgeons at the Columbia-Presbyterian Medical Center invited him to New York to demonstrate his approach to recovery from injuries. In 1938, Hans settled permanently in New York and served for many years on the staff of Columbia-Presbyterian and was also affiliated with Bellevue and Metropolitan hospitals in the city. He also served as an associate professor of physical medicine and rehabilitation at the New York University College of Medicine.

In his private practice, in addition to athletes, patients included Eleanor Roosevelt, Rita Hayworth, Paulette Goddard, Yul Brynner, Angela Lansbury, Arthur Godfrey, Katherine Hepburn, and Lowell Thomas, as well as doormen, cab drivers, bellhops, and cleaning ladies whom he treated at no cost.

Obviously I am a believer in Hans Kraus's approach to injuries. It has worked for me, my family, and thousands of others. But as Hans himself always advised, be sure to consult your own physician before you begin any treatments or exercises discussed in this book because they might not be appropriate for you.

—Robert H. Boyle

Preface

This book has been written for the everyday amateur athlete, such as the housewife who plays tennis several times a week, the businessman or businesswoman who runs every morning before catching the 8:02, the skiing enthusiast, and the weekend golfer, among many others, young and old. The book is the result of years of research and clinical practice in the field of physical medicine and rehabilitation, and it details advances made in that specialty that are unknown to the public at large, most general practitioners and many orthopedic surgeons.

Briefly put, the book shows you how to condition yourself no matter what sport you play, and by so doing improve your performance and guard yourself against injury at the same time. In the event you do suffer injury, both treatment and rehabilitation procedures that will get you back into play as soon as possible are discussed in detail. On a personal note, I can attest to the effectiveness of these procedures both as patient and physician. I have been involved in sports all my life and have suffered my share of injuries, but I have always been able to return to play because I have used these procedures on myself.

It should be noted that several exercises in the book have been intentionally repeated in different chapters for the convenience of the reader.

I would like to thank Dr. Bert Angrist, Mr. Ellis H. Hendrix, RPT (Registered Physical Therapist), Mr. Alexander Melleby, Mr. and Mrs. James P. McCarthy, Mr. and Mrs. Wallace Raubenheimer, and Mr. William Peck for reading the manuscript and making helpful suggestions. I would especially like to thank Dr. Gretchen Besser, who not only reviewed different drafts of the manuscript but went over them, line by line, and word for word. My thanks also to Mrs. Madi Frances Kraus for doing the drawings in the book. Finally, I would like to thank Mr. Robert H. Boyle, who helped edit and prepare the book.

HANS KRAUS, M.D.

THE SPORTS INJURY HANDBOOK

Hans Kraus, M.D.

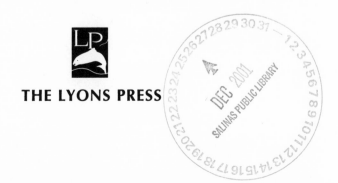

THE LYONS PRESS

Printed in the United States of America

10   9   8   7   6   5   4   3   2   1

The Library of Congress Cataloging-in-Publication Data is available on file.

PART ONE

Prevention Through Fitness and Exercise

1

The Muscular System

You're playing tennis, you're jogging, skiing, swimming, wrestling, playing racket ball, cycling, hiking, climbing, or lifting weights. You're one of the millions of Americans now active in participant sports. It's great to keep yourself in physical and mental trim through vigorous exercise. If you feel that way, good for you, and read on because this book can do a lot to help you avoid injury and to put you at the peak of your abilities. Then again, perhaps you're not feeling so wonderful from all the exercise. You've got that pain in your elbow that won't go away. Or maybe it's shin splints, a hamstring pull that keeps recurring or a nagging twinge in your back. This book is for you, too, because it will show you how to recondition yourself.

An estimated twenty million Americans now hurt themselves each year playing sports. The lame and the sore troop into their doctors' offices every day. "Doctor, just as I hit the ball off the first tee . . ." "When I tried to put backspin on the ball . . ." "I felt the pain in my knee right after I'd run the first mile . . ." "My back went out just as I was getting ready to . . ."

Sound familiar? Of course, but it need not happen to you. After many years in medical practice, first as a fracture surgeon and then as a specialist in physical medicine and rehabilitation, I can assure you that the majority of injuries

3

suffered by amateur athletes should never have occurred in the first place. You don't have to suffer from shin splints, tennis elbow, sprains, strains, charley horses, stiff neck, "runner's knee," pulled hamstrings, muscle spasms, low back pain, or stiff shoulders.

There is no great mystery about such ailments. Some may be caused by faulty movement, such as tennis elbow, which usually occurs because of failure to follow through on the backhand. However, most athletic injuries occur because the muscles are not in condition. There are a lot of injuries simply because there are a lot of people playing sports with muscles that are weak or tight.

How do you know if your muscles are good enough for sports? That's very easy. Take the seven simple Minimum Sports Fitness Tests shown in chapter 2. These tests measure your muscular strength and flexibility, and if you fail even one of them, you're a prime candidate for injury. What do you do then? Instead of playing sports, start the conditioning program as indicated. After you have finished the program, you should be able to pass the seven Minimum Sports Fitness Tests. When you pass, you can start to play sports. If by chance you can't pass those tests but have been playing sports without injury, don't think I'm wrong in calling you a candidate for injury. You're playing on borrowed time, and you're likely to end up in the doctor's office.

If you pass the seven Minimum Sports Fitness Tests the first time you take them, go ahead and play sports. But it is important that you do the exercises recommended in chapter 3 as a warm-up before play and then as a cool-down afterwards. These exercises, which are designed to relax, limber, and stretch your muscles, will help to enhance your performance and guard against injury.

Chapter 5 deals with individual sports. It offers my candid assessment of a number of sports, the physical demands they require or impose, the equipment needed, and advice on how to avoid potential injury problems inherent in different sports. Of course, it is impossible to guarantee that anyone playing sports won't get hurt, but in the event you do, chapters 6 through 11 show you how to recover fully from a sprain, strain, or fracture. You should always bear the following in mind about any athletic injury: the injured part is highly likely to be reinjured if it is not brought back to full strength and flexibility before you play again. This is because the movements in sports are repetitive, and if you play before you are fully recovered, you will subject the injured part to the same trauma that occurred before the injury took place. When you do this, you are not only exposing yourself to reinjury, but you risk making the condition worse. However, if you follow the directions given in chapters 6 through 11, you can restore the injured part to full strength and flexibility and then return to play. You might also be surprised to find out that you can return to play sooner than you might have expected.

YOUR MUSCULAR SYSTEM

If medical practice has lagged anywhere in this country, it is in the failure to keep up with the advances made by specialists in the field of physical medicine and rehabilitation. Medicine has paid too little attention to the muscular system, even though it is of vital importance to personal health. Your muscles allow you to move and express your thoughts. Your use of your muscles affects your metabolism. If you exercise sufficiently, you set up a natural balance against overweight. An athlete in training can consume up to 6,000 calories a day without gaining weight. Vigorous exercise also relaxes both your muscles and your mind. Indeed, fifteen minutes of exercise that causes the heart to beat 100 to 120 times a minute has been shown to have a measurably greater tranquilizing effect than 400 milligrams of meprobamate, the generic name for Miltown and Equanil. By contrast, underexercise has been correlated with muscle pain, obesity, coronary heart disease, duodenal ulcers, diabetes, "tension," and emotional instability.

It may be news to you that your mind can influence your muscles and vice versa, for better or worse, but just take a look at yourself the next time you're irritated or annoyed. What happens, for instance, when another car cuts you off in traffic? You tighten your grip on the wheel and your muscles tense. Any kind of external irritation—a loud record player next door, the whine of a neighbor's chain saw, getting stuck on a broken-down commuter train—can cause muscles to tense. The same goes for internal irritations. Just *thinking* about a personal problem—the next mortgage payment or an impending visit from an annoying relative—can cause your muscles to tense.

Adding to the burden is the fact that living in twentieth-century cities and suburbs doesn't give you a chance to get rid of tension physically because almost everything is mechanized. Our ancestors walked, ran, rode a horse, and drove a carriage whereas we ride in a car, probably with power steering. Instead of plowing fields and bringing in the harvest, we shop at the supermarket. Instead of walking upstairs, we take an elevator. Instead of washing clothes by hand in a tub, we put them in a machine. Even can openers, carving knives, and toothbrushes have become electrified.

As a result of the constant assault of irritations and the inability to work them off in the course of daily living, many persons lead the lives of caged animals. Their muscles become more stiff and tight because they don't work off the accumulated tension. The only way you can work off tension is through purposeful physical exercise, be it tennis, running, weight lifting, or whatever, and then you have to know what you're doing with your muscular system. You just can't run out to play. You have to warm up beforehand and cool down afterwards. Otherwise you can wreak havoc with your muscles. This holds true for professionals as well as amateurs like you, no matter how vigorous you have been physically. Just the other day a tennis pro, who was highly seeded in the U.S. Nationals, had to withdraw because he pulled a hamstring in his first-round match.

How does a muscle work? To produce strength, it shortens and tightens. It becomes tense by contracting, and it performs whatever task you want it to do, such as hitting a ball, bending your knee, or turning your shoulder. After the muscle has performed the task, it normally expands to its initial length and goes into a state of relaxation. It loses its tension while other muscles take over, contract, become tense, do their job, and then let go and return to a state of relaxation. This flow of tensing and relaxing muscles produces the fluid movement that characterizes the performance of the well-conditioned athlete or dancer.

The more you use a muscle, the stronger it becomes. But to function properly, a muscle also has to be flexible, and to be flexible it must relax. Tightness and tension inhibit flexibility of a muscle. Over a period of time, such a muscle becomes shortened, and constantly tense and painful. Let me cite the case of Les B., an energetic man in his late twenties who had taken up running and suddenly suffered from what is popularly called runner's knee in his right leg. In constant pain and unable to run, he went to a physician who injected cortisone. When the pain failed to go away, the physician referred him to an orthopedic surgeon who prescribed strengthening exercises for the knee. Les B. performed the exercises as instructed, but the pain persisted. He was then informed that surgery was necessary and that after the operation he should never run again. Advised to seek another opinion, Les B. hobbled into our clinic. I examined him and took a detailed case history. I told him that surgery was not necessary because the pain in his knee was caused by tight quadriceps. When tense and tight, these thigh muscles direct pain to the knee. He would be able to run again after he did flexibility exercises. The strengthening exercises he had previously done had only made his quadriceps muscles tighter and aggravated the condition. I also advised him to warm up before and cool down after running, to stop running on a hard surface, and to see a podiatrist about getting arch supports. Les B. started doing the flexibility exercises, and in two weeks he was able to resume running. Seven years have now passed and Les B. is still running, and he does so without pain.

A tight muscle is also vulnerable to tear when suddenly stretched. When I speak of a muscle tear, I'm not trying to conjure up a picture of a muscle being ripped in half like a piece of cheesecloth. Most tears of a muscle are so small that they do not produce bleeding, yet they can throw a muscle into spasm.

MUSCLE PAIN

There are many kinds of injuries that an athlete can suffer, but it is important to keep in mind that there are only four different kinds of muscle pain that you can have. If you appreciate the differences, you can treat the pain appropriately. I cannot stress this enough because muscle pain is often baffling to both athlete and physician. The four kinds of muscle pain are:

1. *Pain from muscle spasm.* This occurs following an acute strain, sprain, or fracture. The spasm is caused by painful contraction of the muscle, which sets off a vicious cycle of pain and contraction, pain and contraction. A spasm can endure for days unless it is broken. It can be broken by ethyl chloride spray, which is very effective, ice massage, or in the case of back spasm, by a hot pack. These local measures should be used in conjunction with gentle limbering motion, which is discussed in detail in chapters 6 and 7. Spasm responds poorly to oral pain medication and tranquilizers,

but pain from muscle tension, discussed below, responds well to analgesics and tranquilizers.

2. *Pain from muscle tension.* This pain is caused by a muscle that contracts past the momentary need. Examples are tension headache, tension neck pain, and tension backache. This is the nagging pain that causes you to speak a medical truth when you say, "So-and-so is a pain in the neck" or "So-and-so is a pain in the behind." When a muscle contracts, it produces weak electric currents: the intensity of the currents is in proportion to the degree of muscle contraction. Using electrodes, Drs. Peter Sainsbury and T. G. Gibson in England examined a number of people who complained of habitual tension headaches or muscle pain. One set of electrodes was affixed to the muscle or muscles producing the pain, the "target" areas, and another set was attached to "normal" muscles that did not produce pain. Sainsbury and Gibson then put the subjects through an interview deliberately designed to induce tension. As the interview proceeded, the two physicians discovered that the normal muscles began to tense—though not as much as the target muscles—and then relaxed quickly after the interview. By contrast, the target muscles not only increased in tension during the interview, but their tension increased even more after the interview as the subjects complained of pain. Muscle tension responds to relaxation exercises and to tranquilizers.

3. *Pain from muscle deficiency.* This is caused by weak and/or stiff muscles. The case just cited of Les B. is an example. His stiff quadriceps directed pain to the knee, but he was able to run again after the quadriceps muscle was made flexible through exercise. Another example: weak abdominal muscles that cause low back pain. The classic example of this is the low back pain some mothers suffer after pregnancy. A weak and/or stiff muscle predisposes you to injury. Muscle deficiency responds to therapeutic exercises designed to correct it.

4. *Pain from triggerpoints.* The most neglected of all causes of muscle pain, triggerpoints are small hard nodules in muscle that can literally trigger pain and spasm. They have been biopsied and shown to be areas of degenerated muscle tissue. Max Lange, a German orthopedic surgeon, described the distribution, origin, and pathology of triggerpoints in 1931, and although other researchers have since written about them extensively, most physicians are completely unaware of the existence of triggerpoints and their significance.

Prolonged muscle tension, chronic strain, spasm, or trauma can cause triggerpoints, which most often occur near the insertion of muscle into tendon or bone. For instance, tennis elbow is most often caused by one or more triggerpoints that develop from repeated shock to the forearm muscles from faulty handling of the racket. Similarly, baseball pitchers who suffer from arm or shoulder pain often have triggerpoints because of the repeated strain of throwing a ball. Although triggerpoints can develop in any muscle, they most frequently occur in the neck, shoulder, upper back, lower back, hip, and calf muscles as illustrated here.

When relatively minor episodes of pain caused by triggerpoints go unrecognized and untreated, the episodes of pain will increase in frequency, duration, and intensity, sometimes to the point where the sufferer feels almost permanently disabled. The search for triggerpoints requires careful examination by a physician. The muscles should first be probed with the fingertips because triggerpoints can sometimes be palpated. More often than not, the patient will respond to the physician's probing fingers by wincing and complaining of pain when a tender spot is touched. Certain complaints—shoulder pain, painful neck, occipital headache, back pain, painful calf muscles, runner's knee—are frequently caused by triggerpoints.

The patient should have each triggerpoint treated separately. It is best to let a day go by in between treatment of

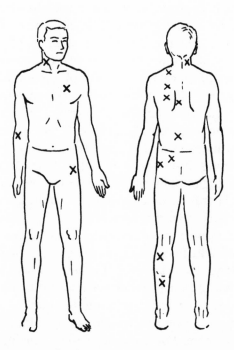

each triggerpoint, which can be eliminated only by mechanical destruction. That isn't as bad as it sounds. Mechanical destruction involves needling with a hypodermic syringe filled with lidocaine. If the patient is sensitive to lidocaine, we use a pure physiological saline solution that matches the salt content of blood. We move the needle around in a circle touching all the soreness in the triggerpoint, at the same time injecting lidocaine with each insertion of the needle. The repetitious needling and the injection of the fluid combine to break up the triggerpoint. In the three to four days after injection, we use electric muscle stimulation, ethyl chloride spray, and gentle exercises to complete treatment of the affected muscle.

On occasion, we see patients who are in muscle spasm induced by triggerpoints. Here it is essential to treat the spasm first and the triggerpoints at a later time.

Sometimes it is possible to relieve the pain from trigger-points temporarily by the application of pressure, but trigger-points can be eliminated only by needling and injection. I know this not only from treating countless patients but from my own personal experience. Once while mountain climbing I had to chin myself with one hand over an overhang. If I hadn't I would have suffered a terrible fall. As I pulled myself over the overhang, I felt something tear in my right shoulder. Although it hurt, I climbed not only that day but for the following three weeks as well. I knew from the pain that I had a triggerpoint in the shoulder-blade muscle, and in self-experiment I decided to see if I could get rid of it by various means. I tried pressure, heat, cold, and electrother-apy. None of these methods worked. Then I had the trigger-point needled and injected, and that finally eliminated it.

Back in 1931 when Lange published his book on trigger-points, he predicted that twenty years would pass before the medical profession recognized their significance and impor-tance. He was an optimist. Even today few standard medical works discuss them. For example, *Taber's Cyclopedic Medi-cal Dictionary*, twelfth edition, 1970, makes no mention whatever of triggerpoints. There is an entry, however, on tennis elbow, which is defined as "an obscure, insidious dis-tressing complaint." According to the dictionary, treatment is as follows: "In mild cases, immobilization by a splint or adhesive strapping, supplemented by heat or diathermy. In long continued cases, surgical intervention may be indi-cated."

It is important to bear in mind that triggerpoints can occur in the well-conditioned athlete. For example, the leg muscles of a distance runner are likely to be stiff for at least a week after a race, and stiff muscles are prone to injury. Take the case of G.B., a young woman who placed high in the Boston Marathon. While out running several days later in the park, she suddenly twisted to the right to avoid a cyclist. She felt some pain in her right hip but continued to run. In the course of the next several days, pain also spread to her right calf and lower back. She went for an examination and was told that she had a disc problem and should rest in bed. She rested in bed for two weeks but failed to improve. She was told to go to bed for three weeks. She did but still did not improve, so she came to see us. We took a complete case history and examined her. Her right hamstring muscles were very tight, and she had triggerpoints in her back, hip, and calf muscles. We began injection and elimination of the triggerpoints and then started her on a program designed to relax and stretch her muscles. After two months of treatment, G.B. resumed running.

One other point should be noted about triggerpoints. They also frequently occur in persons with endocrine imbalance, such as women in menopause or persons suffering from hypothyroidism or Addison's disease.

2

Testing Your Fitness: The Minimum Sports Fitness Test

"On your mark, get set, go!" the starter shouts as the race begins. Are you ready to run five miles, jog two miles, swim 200 yards, or play a hard match in tennis? You think you are? Good for you, but are you sure that you can without hurting yourself? Here is a very easy way to find out if your muscles are in shape for sports. You can test yourself right now by taking the Minimum Sports Fitness Tests shown below. These basic tests are keyed to your body weight. Obviously, if you are grossly overweight, your chances of passing are nil.

If you have back pain, a cardiovascular condition, or any other health problem, check with your physician before taking the tests. Otherwise, they can be taken by anyone. They are designed to show the fitness of your locomotor apparatus and whether or not you have minimum muscular strength and flexibility for sports.

You'll need an assistant to help you with the first test. Before you take the tests make sure you are comfortable. Take off your shoes and strip down to your undergarments. Be at ease. Don't rush. Don't strain. Simply take the tests as directed.

3

Warming Up and Cooling Down: The Sports Fitness Exercise Program

If you have passed all the Minimum Sports Fitness Tests, you are ready to take the Sports Fitness Exercise Program. The dozen exercises in this program will do several things for you. By relaxing and stretching your muscles, the exercises will prepare you for play. They will help safeguard you against injury. They will also help you to unwind or cool down after play. Do exercises 1 through 12 before you play. After you play do the exercises in reverse order, 12 through 1. This daily program will take only ten minutes, five minutes before you play, five minutes afterwards.

Once you start, be sure to do the exercises every day, even if you're not playing, because they will keep your muscles strong and flexible. If you happen to have a very hectic day and are pressed for time, take the time to do the exercises because they will relieve tension caused by the stresses of the day. Stress is the greatest enemy we face, but you can defeat it by doing the exercises.

Do each exercise three times before moving on to the next exercise. Do them slowly and smoothly. Don't strain, don't push, don't do jerky movements. Be sure to rest for a second between each exercise, and also between each set of exercises. Do as many sets as you feel up to on the first day, but avoid tiring yourself. Fatigue can lead to soreness and stiffness. Take it easy. If you are strong but tense, you may try to do the exercises too quickly. Pace yourself. Again, take it easy. Make yourself comfortable. Take off your shoes and strip down to your underclothes. You're now ready to begin.

Exercise 1

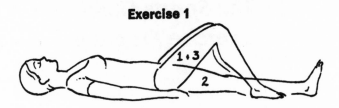

Position yourself comfortably on your back on the floor with both knees bent. Close your eyes. Take a deep breath and exhale slowly. Slide your right leg forward and slide it back. Slide the left leg forward and slide it back. Take another deep breath. Tighten both fists, then let go.

Exercise 2

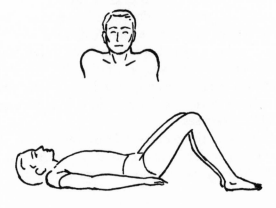

Take a deep breath, then exhale slowly. Now shrug and breathe in. Exhale as you let go of the shrug.

Exercise 3

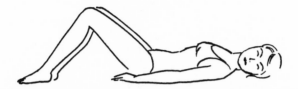

Turn your head all the way to the left, then return it to the normal front-and-center position and relax. Turn your head all the way to the right, as far as you can, return to normal position, and relax.

Exercise 4: Double Knee Flex

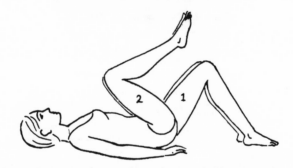

Still on your back, flex both knees. Pull both knees up to your chest. Then lower your legs gradually to the floor in the flexed position. Do not raise your hips off the floor.

Exercise 5: Cat Back

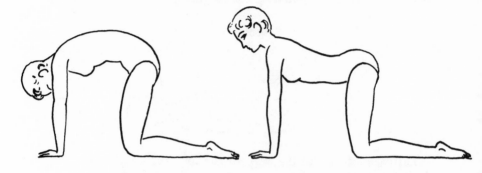

Assume a kneeling position, resting on your hands and knees. Arch your back like a cat and drop your head at the same time. Now reverse the arch by bringing up your head and forming a U with your spine.

Exercise 6: Pectoral Stretch

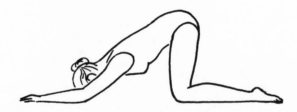

From a kneeling position, place your hands, then your forearms on the floor. Gradually straighten your back, sliding forward on your arms and keeping your back and head straight. This will stretch your pectoral muscles as you move away from your knees. Return to a kneeling position by walking back up with your arms. Thighs are always perpendicular to the floor.

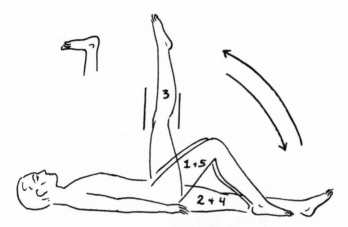

Lie on your back, knees flexed, and slide your right leg out, pointing the toes away from your head. Lock the knee and raise your leg as high as you can without bending. Lower the straight leg to floor and slide it to bent position. Do same for the left leg. Repeat this exercise with heel instead of toe pointing up.

Exercise 10: Hamstring Stretch

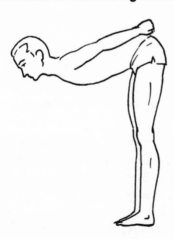

Stand up with heels together and clasp your hands behind your back, keeping your back and neck straight. Bend for-

ward from the hips, gradually lower your trunk, and go
down as far as you can, raising your head until you feel
stretching in the back of your legs.

Exercise 11: Calf Muscle Stretch

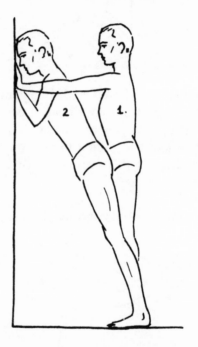

Stand a little bit less than arm's length away from the wall
with feet together. Keep hips and back straight and place
hands flat on wall. Bending your elbows and using your
forearms, slowly allow your straight body to come close to
the wall. Then straighten your arms to push your body to the
standing position. Always keep your hands in contact with
the wall and heels in touch with the floor when leaning into
the wall.

Exercise 12: Floor Touch

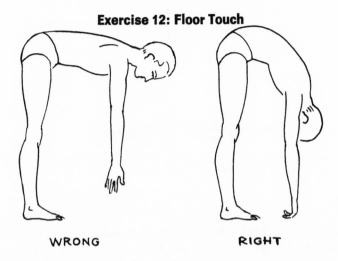

WRONG   RIGHT

This is the peak exercise. Keep your heels together. Relax by inhaling and exhaling deeply. Drop your neck gradually and let your trunk "hang" loosely from your hips. Drop your shoulders and then your back gradually. Let gravity help you. Do this two or three times. When you're completely relaxed and "hanging from the hips," slowly reach down as far as you can without straining. Once you've reached as far as you can, hold the position for a count of three. Now relax again and straighten up.

These are the dozen exercises you do before play. Remember to do each exercise three times before moving on to the next. After you have finished play, do the exercises in reverse order, 12 through 1, again doing each exercise three times. Chapter 5 describes the warm-up exercises you can do for your legs and arms, depending on which sport you play, while the next chapter describes a weight-training program that is optional.

4

Weight Training

Training with light weights can be a useful adjunct to the Sports Fitness Exercise Program no matter what sports you play. This weight-training program is best done on a day when you're not playing sports and you can give it time. Start the weight-training exercises after you have done the first half (exercises 1 through 12) of the Sports Fitness Exercise Program. When you have finished with weight training, then do the Sports Fitness Exercise Program in reverse order as previously described.

You will need to use dumbbells, barbells, and weight boots. Select weights that you can lift easily. That is the key to the program. Later you may add weight that you can handle with your growing strength, so select dumbbells and barbells with removable plates so you can increase weight. When you get to a lift that is too difficult, decrease the weight accordingly. A weight will be too difficult if you cannot lift it clean, that is, go through full range smoothly without jerking.

Normally, weights are lifted in repetitions of ten. If your muscles tend to be stiff, you'll be better off lifting a weight only three or four times before proceeding to the next exercise. If you wish, you may repeat the whole sequence of exercises several times in one session. But stop if you feel tired or cannot perform the movements smoothly.

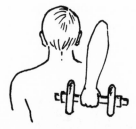

6. Stand up, hold a dumbbell in your right hand, and put it over your right shoulder behind your neck. Return to normal position. Now do the same with the left hand.

STRENGTHENING THE LOWER EXTREMITIES

You will need weight-lifting boots or shot bags. Of special advantage are the "drop foot" weight boots sold by orthopedic supply houses. These boots have an extension to the back of the calf and are strapped to the calf and foot. The weights are attached to a bar that goes across the bottom of the boot, and the boots are very stable.

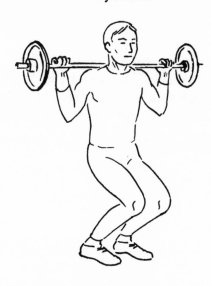

1. Do knee bends with the barbell on your shoulders. Don't force this. Quit at the first sign of fatigue. Too many knee bends with a heavy weight can damage the knees.

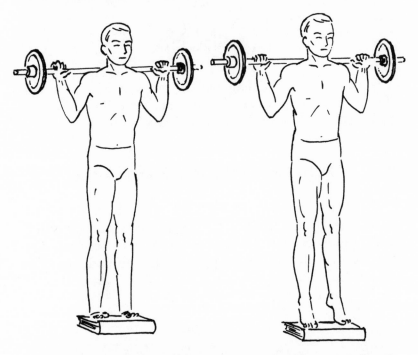

2. Put a book on the floor. With the barbell on your shoulders, put your toes on the book and your heels on the floor. Stand up on your toes, then go back down on your heels. Don't do this exercise if your calf muscles cannot do it easily without the weight.

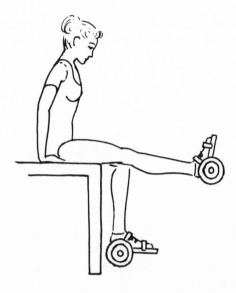

3. Put on the weight boots and sit on the edge of a table. Extend your right leg, then let it hang down again. Do the same with the left leg and relax. Gradually increase the weight, alternating each leg as you exercise.

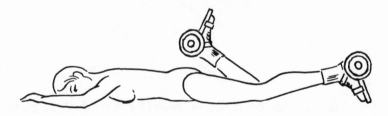

4. Lie on your stomach with your weight boots on. Bring your right heel toward your seat and then relax. Do the same with the left heel.

STRENGTHENING ABDOMINAL MUSCLES

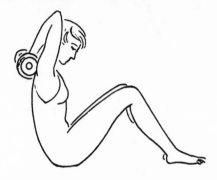

1. Hold a dumbbell in each hand, put your hands behind your neck, and do three sit-ups. You have to be in good shape to do this, and you have to be able to do sit-ups without weights with ease.

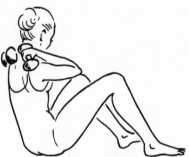

2. Lie on your back, knees flexed, a dumbbell in each hand behind your neck. Sit up, bringing the right elbow to the left knee. Then lie back, and relax. Sit up, bringing the left elbow to the right knee, lie back, and relax.

5

Sports and Activities

After you have done the first half of the Sports Fitness Exercises given in chapter 3, you may want to add the following exercises as part of your warm-up before playing.

If you run, ski, skate, cycle, or engage in any activity involving strenuous use of your legs, sit on the edge of a chair, hold your legs straight out and kick each one rapidly as though swimming. Do this 50 to 100 times. If you have not been very active recently, do this 25 times the first day, 30 the second day, and so on. If you play tennis, squash, or handball, or engage in any activity involving strenuous arm and shoulder movement, do the following warm-ups as well. Swing your arms backward and forward 50 to 100 times, as though you were warming yourself on a cold day. If you haven't been very active recently, do each set of arm swings 25 times the first day and then increase gradually. Additional warm-ups and other exercises for various sports are discussed in this chapter.

JOGGING AND RUNNING

I go along with the saying that jogging is doing a mile in eight minutes or more, while running is doing a mile in seven minutes or less. But no matter whether you jog, run, or sprint, you have to approach running the right way.

In a recent book on sports medicine, an orthopedist wrote that it was pure nonsense for even someone who was totally out of shape to exercise before jogging because jogging is a warm-up in itself. That's wrong. Jogging is *not* a warm-up at all. You must do relaxing, limbering, and stretching exercises before and after you jog because otherwise your muscles will tighten up. Running does a lot for you, but it does not do everything, and you must supplement it with relaxing and stretching exercises.

Some people get a tremendous "high" when they run, while others find running boring. If you get a high when you run, take care that you don't become addicted to running to the point where it is the be-all and end-all to life. Keep your running under control, don't let it dominate you. If you find running boring, that is all to the good physiologically. Let me explain. For example, tennis is not boring. A match is exciting, and while you're playing, you work off the tensions induced by the game itself. But the problem with tennis is, how much more physical activity do you have to do to work off the other tensions of the day? And that's why running is valuable if you find it boring. It has no tensions of its own, so you can work off the stress of the day.

If you're going to run, make sure you're in shape to do so. Did you pass the Minimum Sports Fitness Tests? If you didn't, don't run until you can, particularly if you failed the floor-touch test. There are any number of people who start running, like it, but then have to quit because they suffer pain, usually in the legs or the lower back. They haven't suffered any injury per se, but they have pain for one or both of two reasons: they weren't in shape to start running, and/or they failed to do relaxing and stretching exercises. Running a mile requires about 1,750 footfalls, and that puts stress on the lower extremities and the lower back muscles.

STRENGTHENING THE UPPER EXTREMITIES

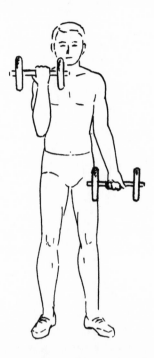

1. Alternate Curl. With palms up and dumbbells in both hands, bring your right hand to your shoulder, then lower it. Now lift a dumbbell to your left shoulder and lower it.

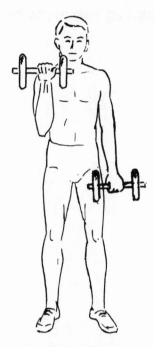

2. Alternate Reverse Curl. With palms down and dumbbells in both hands, do the same movements as in the previous exercise.

A woman should be able to do three modified chins. Place a broomstick between two chairs, lie flat on the floor, and pull yourself up three times.

Minimum Sports Fitness Test No. 6, Man

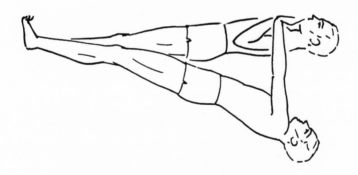

A man should be able to do three push-ups.

Minimum Sports Fitness Test No. 6, Woman

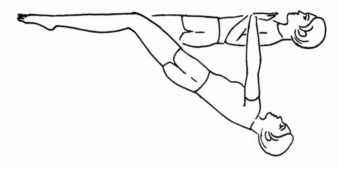

A woman should be able to do three modified push-ups. Lie flat on your stomach on the floor. Now push up, keeping your knees on the floor.

Minimum Sports Fitness Test No. 5, Man

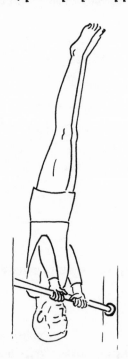

A man should be able to do three chins.

Minimum Sports Fitness Test No. 5, Woman

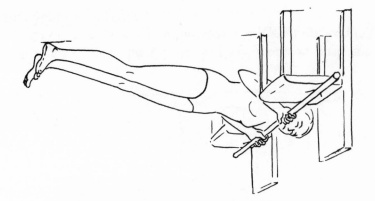

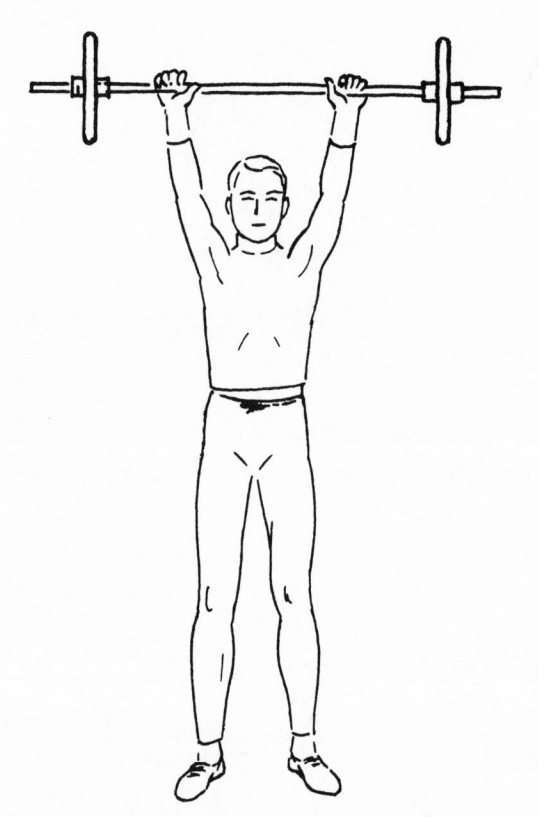

3. Overhead Press. Standing, lift the barbell overhead from your chest.

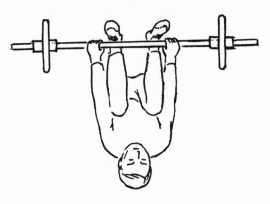

4. Military Press. With your knees flexed, lift barbell from the floor and bring it to your chest. Now raise it over your head and lower it to the floor.

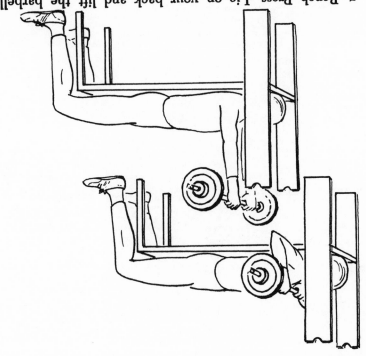

5. Bench Press. Lie on your back and lift the barbell straight up over your chest, then lower it.

Exercise 8: Hamstring Stretch

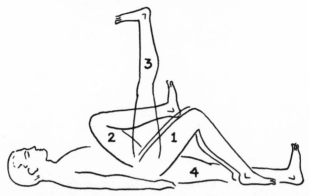

To do exercise 8, lie on your back with both knees flexed, arms at sides. Bring right knee up as close as possible to your chest, extend your right leg, pointing the toes toward the ceiling. Keeping the knee straight, lower your leg to the floor. Then slide the leg back up to the bent position. Do the same for the left leg.

Now do the exercise with the heel pointing up toward the ceiling. This stretches the soleus muscle in the back of the calf, while the previous exercise stretches the gastrocnemius muscle in the front of the calf.

Exercise 9: Hamstring Stretch

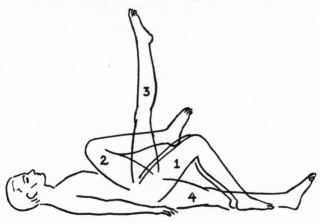

Exercise 7: Sit-up, Knees Flexed

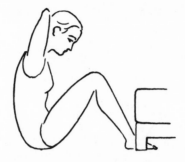

Lie on your back with your hands clasped behind your neck, knees flexed. Tuck your feet under a heavy object that won't topple (a chest of drawers, bed, or heavy chair, for example). Sit up, then lower yourself slowly to a lying position. You should sit up gradually, first by raising your head, then your shoulders, and then your chest and lower end of the spine. Do not sit up by holding your trunk stiff and jerking your weight up. If you cannot do this exercise with your hands behind your neck, try to do it with your hands at your sides. Later, cross them over your stomach, and still later, when you are stronger, bring your crossed arms up to your chest and, finally, behind your neck and head. If you're unable to do this exercise at all, continue with the earlier exercises until you have gained enough strength to manage this one. Before each sit-up take a deep breath and exhale as you curl to a sit-up position.

Minimum Sports Fitness Test No. 3

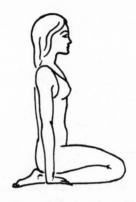

Get on your knees and sit back on your heels.

Minimum Sports Fitness Test No. 4

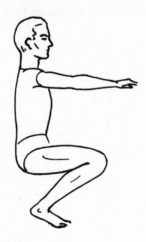

Do three knee bends.

If you use your arms in sports such as skiing or tennis, you should be able to pass the following tests, depending on whether you are a man or a woman.

Minimum Sports Fitness Test No. 1

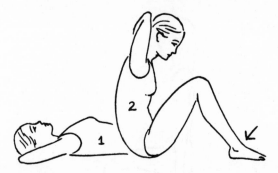

Lie on your back on the floor with your hands clasped behind your neck. Flex your knees. Have your assistant hold your ankles down. Now roll up into a sitting position. This tests the strength of your abdominal muscles.

Minimum Sports Fitness Test No. 2

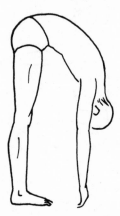

Stand up straight with your legs together. Slowly lean over and reach down as far as you can. If your muscles are sufficiently flexible, you should be able to touch the floor with ease with your fingertips. *Do not force this movement or bob. This may cause backstrain.*

you think you are. It's like racing a car without an adequate chassis. Sooner or later something is bound to break down. Moreover, you're not getting as much out of your sport as you should or could because your muscles are deficient. I'll give you an example. I know a very good athlete, a marathon runner named Rick G. He did very well competitively, although he suffered from thigh and back pain after every race. He tested himself and he couldn't touch the floor with his fingertips because his hamstrings were tight. These tight muscles caused the pain. As a result he enrolled in the Y's Way to a Healthy Back program which I had designed for the YMCA. Besides alleviating back problems, this exercise program, which is given in full in chapter 10, is an excellent muscular conditioner. Rick stayed in the Y's program for three months until he could touch the floor with his fingertips. By then, the thigh and back pain had disappeared. Moreover, when Rick resumed running, he bettered his own times because he had lengthened his stride as the result of stretching his hamstrings.

Minimum Sports Fitness Test No. 7, Either Sex

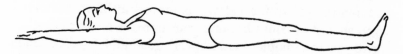

Lie on your back on the floor. Now extend your arms back so that your elbows are straight and the backs of your arms touch the floor.

If you pass all these tests, it means that you have sufficient muscular strength and flexibility to play sports. But remember, these are *minimum* tests. To guard against injury and to improve your showing in sports, do the basic sports exercise program described in chapter 3. Depending on what sport you play, also do the special exercises given in the same chapter.

If you have failed any one of the Minimum Sports Fitness Tests, you're not ready to play sports without risking injury. If you failed test No. 1, do exercise 7 in chapter 3. If you failed test No. 2, do exercises 1–4 in chapter 3, then gradually add others until you are doing the full program. Do not play sports until you can do exercise 12 with ease. If you failed test No. 3, do exercise 4 described at the end of the entry on jogging and running in chapter 5. If you failed test No. 4, do exercise 3 described under the heading of strengthening the lower extremities in chapter 4. If you failed tests Nos. 5–6, do exercises 1–6 for strengthening the upper extremities in chapter 4. If you failed test No. 7, do exercises 1–3, 6, and 10 for shoulder strain or sprain in chapter 8. Although these exercises are for an injured shoulder, they work equally well for shoulders with stiff muscles.

If it happens that you couldn't pass all these tests but yet have been playing without suffering injury or pain, don't scoff. You have been playing on borrowed time, and you are a prime candidate for injury, no matter how good an athlete

I recommend running very highly. It will give your cardio-vascular system a good workout and it will keep your body trim, especially if you're in middle age. Men in their forties tend to put on weight with a potbelly while women get the weight in their behinds.

Like all good things, running can be carried to excess. It is ironic, but for years I used to preach the value of vigorous sports and exercise to a sedentary America. Now we're in the midst of a sports explosion, and too many people are carry-ing things to an extreme. I have the marathon particularly in mind. The country is now in the grip of a marathon mania. I use the word mania because many people are simply not equipped physically to cope with the stresses that the mara-ton imposes. In the past few years, I have had an increas-ing number of marathon runners come to me with ankle problems, knee problems, fatigue fractures, and other injuries brought on by continuous and prolonged pounding on pave-ment. The human foot is not built to run on completely hard and unresilient surfaces for very long distances using iden-tical repetitive movements. If you're running in a marathon or planning to do so, do yourself a favor and think about it. Wouldn't you do better to cut back to a five- or ten-mile race?

If you are going to run, here are some basic points to fol-low. First of all, get a checkup by a good internist. If you're in good health, then have your feet examined by a compe-tent podiatrist. Very few feet are perfect, and feet that are adequate for walking may not hold up for running.

Make sure that you have shoes that are good for your feet. The shoe should bend easily at the ball. A shoe that is stiff at the ball can cause tightening of the calf muscles. Avoid a shoe with a narrow heel. A narrow heel is unstable and can cause ankle sprain. Ankle sprain can also be caused by a shoe with an unusually soft sole. Although an ultrasoft sole would appear to absorb shock, it allows the foot to sink in unevenly and the ankle to wobble.

If your foot has a high arch, it is likely to be relatively rigid with joint ranges less than average. According to Dr. Richard O. Schuster, a leading podiatrist, a high-arched foot is usually associated with a tight calf muscle and a tight long plantar ligament that runs from the heel to the metatarsal bones. A high-arched foot also has a relatively small weight-bearing pattern, and is susceptible to heel pains, pressure concentrations, impact shock, and other painful conditions. As Dr. Schuster says, "The high-arched foot requires flexibility exercises, particularly for the short calf muscle. It functions best in a running shoe with a heel that is considerably thicker than the sole."

A runner with a high-arched foot does better at shorter than longer distances, while the reverse appears to be true for the runner with a low arch. The low-arched foot is usually more flexible and the joint ranges are more than average. Pressure concentrations and impact shock are less of a problem because the low-arched foot has a relatively large weight-bearing pattern.

More often than not, a person with flat feet will need orthotics in the running shoes. Prolonged standing, hiking, but most of all running will cause trouble for the foot, leg, and even the back. We see many cases of back pain produced by prolonged running or standing on flat feet. Similarly, a pronated heel, that is, a heel tilted outward and not perpendicular to the Achilles tendon, may cause foot, leg, or back problems for a runner. This holds true even for minor pronation unless proper supports are used.

Uphill running can be very stressful for runners with short calf muscles, tight Achilles tendons, and tight plantar ligaments. Downhill running can be very stressful for runners with knee problems. Dr. Schuster says, "Balancing foot devices plus extra heel lifts are helpful in these situations."

Recently I saw a young woman, Helen S., who had pain in her left knee. She had taken up running six months before, and she soon had pain. She had the knee examined and was informed it had a loose patella. She was also told not to run anymore. She came to us for a second opinion. Our examination revealed no loose patella in the knee. Instead, Helen S. had flat feet, a heel that flared out, and a slight case of knock-knee. Moreover, her left leg was a quarter inch longer than her right leg. In running, the longer leg is more likely to suffer injury first. (An eighth-inch difference in leg length doesn't mean much, but a difference of a quarter inch or more can cause difficulties.) All these factors had combined to produce stress and pain in the knee. Thanks to therapy, a daily exercise program, and a new pair of corrective running shoes, Helen S. resumed running in six weeks without any recurrence of pain. Knee pain and groin pain are frequent occurrences in runners who have foot problems or who do not do stretching exercises in their warm-ups.

Make sure you're warmed up properly before you jog or run. Do the relaxing, stretching, and kicking exercises. Jog a little bit, stop, jog a little bit again. You'll know that you're warmed up enough to begin serious jogging or running when you break into a light sweat. Without a good warm-up, you expose yourself to possible hamstring or calf-muscle tears. Some years ago, I suddenly began seeing a number of sprinters who came to our clinic for treatment of hamstring or calf-muscle tears. All were from the same university, and had spent only about five minutes warming up. When a sixth sprinter from the same school came in with a hamstring tear, I decided to call the coach, a very senior figure in track circles. I told the coach, "Five or ten minutes is not enough time for a sprinter to warm up. Your boys have to be hot and sweating before they run." I also impressed upon the coach the need for relaxing and stretching exercises. To all this, the coach just said, "Thanks." After that we didn't get any more sprinters from the school, and I thought that the coach was angry at me for daring to tell him what to do. A couple of years later, when I was giving a talk at a luncheon for college track coaches, I spoke about the need for a good warm-up. Suddenly a hand shot up in the audience. It was the coach. I thought that he was going to raise hell with me. Instead he said, "I can attest to what the doctor is saying. A couple of years ago I sent some sprinters with torn hamstrings to his clinic. He called me up and said they weren't warming up properly. After that I never sent another boy to that clinic. I didn't have to because I saw to it that the boys worked up a sweat and relaxed and stretched before they ran."

When you run, use your foot properly. A sprinter runs on the forefoot, but a jogger or long-distance runner goes heel and toes. You land on the heel, go over to the toes, and push off the toes. If you run a distance on your toes, you risk trouble with your calf muscles.

I must emphasize this point: avoid jogging or running on a hard surface, such as cement or asphalt. A lot of city joggers run on hard pavement, and they get into difficulty because of this. Running on a hard surface can produce the same undesirable results that occur if you run when you are tense. You'll get a pain in the calf muscle when it tightens up. Then you'll get pain in the hip muscles, and finally the back muscles. Running on a hard surface can also cause shin splints or stress fractures. Avoid running on unusually soft or loose surfaces. Running on loose sand causes the heels to sink, and this can cause problems with the Achilles tendon and leg muscles. Also avoid running on small tracks that have fifteen turns or more to the mile. They are steeply banked, so that you are forced to run on a slant. As a result, the impact does not go straight up, and you can strain a knee or an ankle. You can also develop groin pain or chondromalacia of the patella (softening of the cartilage in the kneecap).

If you're new to jogging, start off easily. Don't push it. After doing the first half of your Sports Fitness Exercise

Program and warming up, walk a short stretch. Then jog, but stop before you tire. Resume walking, jog a short stretch again, and stop. Lie down and do the second half of your exercise program. Build up your distance gradually. Run every day, but if that is impossible, run not less than three days a week. And to repeat a point I can't stress enough, always make sure to do your exercises every day before and after running.

If you are seriously trying to better your running performance, here are four extra exercises you can add to your daily program.

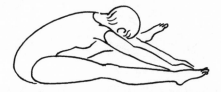

1. Sit with legs apart; reach over and touch both hands to the toes of the right foot. Sit up. Now do the same, touching the left foot.

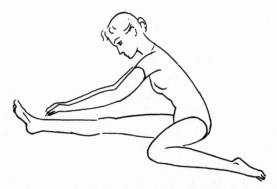

2. Sit in a "hurdle seat," with your right leg extended as though you were hurdling a fence. Touch the toes of the right foot with the right hand and then the left hand. Reverse your seat and do the same with the left foot.

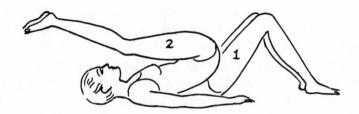

3. Lie on your back, knees bent. Bring both feet way behind your head in a curl.

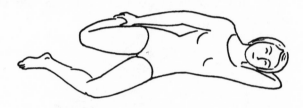

4. Lie on your left side, legs bent. Grasp your right ankle and stretch the thigh muscle by bending the knee as far back as you can. Now lie on your right side and do the same thing with your left ankle.

HIKING AND WALKING

Much of what I have written about running and jogging can be applied to hiking and speed walking. Too much walking can bring on shin splints and even fatigue fractures or stress in the short bones of the foot or the long bones of the leg. Be sure to wear good, sturdy shoes that reach above the ankle and have a firm sole. Never hike in low-cut shoes. You'll be risking ankle injury.

If you're going to walk on a regular basis, start off with easy distances over flat terrain. Then start hiking in hilly or mountainous country. Speed walking or hiking at a brisk pace (five miles an hour) uphill or with a pack will do a good deal not only for your muscles but for your cardiovascular system as well. Indeed, any sport or pastime that involves brisk walking or running, be it beagling or chasing butterflies, is excellent for you.

TENNIS AND RACKET SPORTS

If you play tennis or any other racket sport, be sure to warm up your legs as well as the upper extremities before you play. Lack of a good warm-up can cause tears in the calf muscles, hamstrings, and back muscles. Be wary of the hard-surface tennis court. Hard courts are easy to keep up, but they're not easy on you. Check your shoes and get supports if necessary. You may be better off playing with high shoes rather than low shoes to give your ankles support. The sudden stops, twists, and turns in tennis make you vulnerable to sprained ankle, partial tear of knee ligaments, and injuries to the meniscus (cartilage) in the knee.

Any of the racket sports can produce tennis elbow, but the condition is much rarer in squash, paddle tennis, and racket ball than it is in tennis because of the lighter rackets. Tennis elbow is usually caused by flipping the wrist in an attempt to put top spin on the ball or by failing to follow through on the backhand. A player who fails to follow through slams the emergency brakes on the forearm muscles, so to speak, and this sudden braking puts the muscles under a strain. Repetition produces chronic strain and eventually the development of one or more triggerpoints in the extensor and supinator muscles close to their insertion at the prominent bone of the elbow. A player who persists in playing with tennis elbow sometimes attempts to compensate for the condition by placing greater strain on the upper arm and shoulder, and can end up with additional triggerpoints in the shoulder girdle. Any triggerpoints, of course, must be eliminated by needling and injection. It is also important that the patient consult a coach to learn the proper handling of the racket. Recently, a young man suffering from tennis elbow came to see us, and a week after treatment he was playing again. A month later he was back again with the same problem. He had not taken the coaching lesson we advised, and he had reverted to flipping his wrist on the backhand. This time treatment took two weeks, and then he had the good sense to see a coach.

Tennis elbow isn't confined to persons who play racket sports. We treated a violinist who had tennis elbow in his left arm. By forcing his ear down to the violin, he produced tightness and tenderness down the arm, which resulted in a triggerpoint in the forearm. Other victims of tennis elbow included a man who had to use a screwdriver on his job. Another patient suffering from tennis elbow was fifty years old and very portly. He didn't play tennis, he didn't play the violin, and he rarely used a screwdriver.

"Do you do any physical activity at all?" I asked.

"Not a bit," he said. "I just sit behind a desk all day."

We treated him for a triggerpoint in the forearm, and he was fine in a couple of weeks. A month later he was back with triggerpoint trouble. We treated him again. A month after this, he was back yet again.

"You must do something to produce this triggerpoint," I said.

"I told you, Doctor, I do nothing," he said. "I sit behind a desk all day."

I said, "Okay, sit behind mine, pretend it's yours and show me what you do at work."

He sat down, reached behind, and brought his right hand to his ear.

"What are you doing?" I asked.

"I'm pretending I'm taking a phone call," he said. "I have a phone on a table behind my desk."

I could see why he was getting tennis elbow. Every time he reached for the phone, he strained his forearm. I told him,

"Put the phone on your desk in front of you." This simple advice prevented him from getting tennis elbow again.

One way to guard against tennis elbow is to wear a thumb-lock wristlet, obtainable at an orthopedic supply store. It should be of good, strong material, about two inches wide, and have a Velcro end so it can be adjusted to fit around the wrist, and a loop for the thumb. You put the band on by slipping the thumb through the loop. The loop is anchored

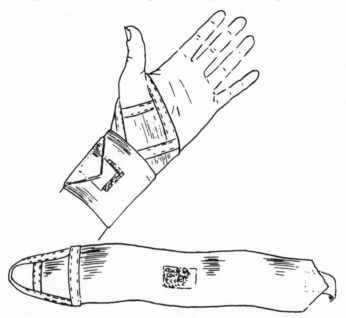

around the thumb and then the band is wrapped around the wrist. This immobilizes the wrist so that you can't flip it easily. Then place an armband around the arm just below the elbow. This prevents the forearm muscles from pulling at the insertion where they join the bone.

You don't have to suffer from a triggerpoint to get a pain in the elbow. Just the other day a psychiatrist I know came to see me with his arm in a brace. He explained that he suffered a sudden pain in his elbow two days earlier after playing tennis. He immediately went to an orthopedist who told him that he had muscle tears near the elbow that might require surgery. The orthopedist put on the brace, but when the pain persisted the psychiatrist came to see me. I removed the brace, sprayed the painful area with ethyl chloride, and he was immediately pain free. He simply had suffered a muscle spasm which was broken by the ethyl chloride.

Persons who play handball, racket ball, and squash are subject to much the same kind of injuries that can afflict tennis players. If you play handball, racket ball, or squash, wear goggles to protect the eyes. Squash is a very fast game, and I see a fair number of players who have suffered acute back pain. Generally they're executives who are tense to start with before they play because of the pressures of the business day. In a hurry to play, they compound the problem by failing to exercise and warm up beforehand.

In handball and all racket sports, special attention should be paid to the upper extremities. Here are three arm exercises you can add to your basic program.

1. Clasp your hands behind your neck. Bring the elbows as far back as possible, then relax.

2. Join your hands behind your back. Bring your arms back as far as possible, then relax.

3. Join your hands as if in prayer and intertwine the fingers. Turn palms out, stretch out the arms, then relax.

SKIING

Skiing is an exhilarating sport, but in the past twenty years it has literally gone downhill. You no longer warm up by clambering uphill; instead you ride a chair lift. Given the time spent standing in line and then riding the lift, you're cold when you start your run and your body really isn't prepared to do the twists and turns necessary, much less to react to an emergency.

Then again, skiing is a seasonal sport, and there are many skiers who don't do anything in the warmer months for physical exercise. It's important that you keep your body in condition during the off months. Lack of proper physical conditioning and lack of skill are two main causes of injury in skiing. There are some people skiing who shouldn't be skiing at all, but with chair lifts going right to the top, skiing has become the sport for many people who are poorly conditioned and/or overweight. Perhaps the latter believe that gravity works in their favor going downhill. I recall a friend of mine who runs a ski school at a resort saying that she had to reject beginners who did not have enough strength to get up on their own after they fell down. I thought she was exaggerating until I went there to ski and saw a couple of students who were unable to raise themselves from the ground, even when they were in correct position to do so.

Anyone who skis, downhill, cross-country, touring, or whatever, is asking for injury unless he or she is in fit condition. If you want to ski, you should be able to do the following exercises with ease.

1. Do six knee bends.
2. Sit back on your heels when kneeling.
3. Run up and down four flights of stairs without feeling strain in your legs.

To prepare yourself for skiing, do push-ups to strengthen your arm extensors, and do a lot of the stretching exercises shown in chapter 3 for the calf muscles, hamstrings, and quadriceps. Do all the stair-walking you can. A friend of mine used to do at least twenty-eight flights of stairs a day. His office was on the fourteenth floor, and he walked up and down instead of taking the elevator. For security reasons the doors are now locked inside the stairwell, so he conditions himself for skiing with uphill and downhill jogging. If you want to build up the strength of your legs and arms for

skiing or any other sport, do the weight exercises given in
this chapter.

Studies of ski injuries underline the importance of physical
conditioning. The members of a Westchester, New York, ski
club skied a total of 5,000 days for eleven years. During that
time, the members had to take part in a preski conditioning
program. No fractures and only two mild sprains occurred.
The next year, the club gave up the conditioning program
and three fractures occurred. At a school in Lake Placid,
New York, fifty children, from eight to fourteen years of age,
accumulated a total of 5,000 skiing hours. Seven fractures
and five sprains occurred. When the school adopted a conditioning program, none of the children in the program suffered accidents in the next 5,000 skiing hours, but two boys
who did not take the program suffered leg fractures. It's also
a fact that injuries rarely occur in ski schools. For instance, at
the Mount Mansfield Ski School in Vermont, only one fracture occurred in 7,310 hours of instruction, while several
Swiss schools reported only one accident in 3,498 hours of
instruction.

Ski equipment can pose a problem. Good release bindings
should prevent many injuries, but they don't necessarily. The
old skis broke, which made up for the fact that they did not
have release bindings. In the old days, I broke a dozen skis
over the years, which probably saved me from a dozen
fractures.

Modern downhill ski boots can cause problems. Last winter, John L., a computer analyst in his late thirties, came
to see me because of a persistent pain in his right knee and a
sore calf muscle. He was at a loss to explain the pain and
soreness. He had never injured the leg, he was in good condition physically, he skied downhill every weekend, and in
the warmer months he played tennis. I asked him to tell me
when he first noticed the condition. "Last Sunday night
when I was driving back home from Vermont," he said. "I
skied all day Saturday and Sunday. The drive back takes

several hours, and as I was driving along I began feeling this pain in the knee. I also felt this soreness in my calf muscle. I came to see you to find out what's wrong, and what I can do about it."

I examined his leg and asked him what kind of ski boots he wore. He told me. They were a very expensive pair of downhill racing boots.

"They're not rear-entry boots, are they?" I asked.

"No, they're not," he said. "Why do you ask?"

I explained. "Modern high, rigid plastic boots are designed to force you into a forward lean with your knees flexed. They're fine for skiing but terrible for standing. They're impossible to walk in, and after you've worn them all day, it's difficult to straighten up. If you wear more common front-entry boots, it's possible to unfasten them at lunchtime or when you're standing in a lift line, so that you can periodicially straighten your knee. In your case, you wore your boots for two days in a row, and then you began to feel pain and soreness on the drive home. The knee reacted because it had been forced into a bend, and the calf muscle became sore because it's also a knee muscle and could not relax." I prescribed exercises for the knee and suggested he buy rear-entry boots that he could open as needed.

It's true there are fewer ankle injuries nowadays than there used to be. With high rigid boots, the accident site has shifted higher. We find more knee injuries and more fractures of the tibia and fibula—the so-called "boot-top." Skiers who wear rigid plastic boots without removing or unfastening them are prime candidates for chronic knee and calf pain. In any case, you should take extra care to limber and stretch your muscles before and after skiing.

I'm very fond of cross-country skiing, which I regard as the best sport of all. It strengthens your arms and legs, it gives you a good cardiovascular workout, and releases tension. At the start of each winter, I always used to cross-country ski before going downhill. Cross-country really got me in condition. By doing this, everything was in balance, and my body was prepared. Unfortunately, most resorts no longer allow uphill walking for safety reasons, and so I suggest doing warm-up exercises before you leave your lodge in the morning.

CYCLING

Like skiing, cycling has fallen victim to fashion, and the vogue is for ten-speed racing bikes. But because of the low placement of the handlebars, many cyclists come up with stiff necks and painful backs. If this happens to you, consider shifting from racing-type handlebars to handlebars that permit you to maintain an upright position so that your neck is not forced into hyperextension and your back is not bent forward severely. Check the angle of the seat as well. Also check the seat for comfort. Racing bikes have narrow seats that are not comfortable for the average recreational cyclist.

Cycling can be good exercise, but there is one other point to watch. Make sure that you stretch your calf muscles and hamstrings before and after you ride. You should do this because you never extend the full length of your legs when you pedal, and if you don't stretch the calf muscles, hamstrings, and quadriceps, they will shorten up in time. It also helps to raise the seat so you get nearly full reach with your legs, but you still need to do the stretching exercises. Remember also that when you pedal quickly to go fast, you never extend your knees completely. In short, cycling is good exercise but it has to be supplemented by leg exercises before and after.

GOLF

Without question, golf is one of the worst games you can play, but if it's the one activity that gives you pleasure, then play it. Be sure, however, to bear the following in mind so you don't fool yourself into thinking that the game does a lot for you physically.

First of all, forget the idea that golf is relaxing. It is not. It is stimulating. The tension it builds can reach extraordinary heights with just one missed putt. The mental strains of golf cause your muscles to tighten. However, you don't work off the tension in your muscles, because golf is not at all demanding physically. You don't run when you golf. In all likelihood you don't even walk but ride in a cart. Even if you were to walk, the slow pace inherent in the game does nothing for your body. Golf has become a game for the sedentary. When the United States Golf Association held the first U.S. Senior Open in 1980 for golfers fifty-five or older, some competitors complained that carts were not allowed. Mind you, these players were not typical duffers. They were outstanding professionals and amateurs who were supposed to be at the top of their game, whatever their age.

Golf has become the sport of those who need it least, harried middle-aged executives. They go out to play under the wrong impression that they're going to relax. Instead they wind up with bad backs or golf elbow. Sometimes they may hurt their backs on the course, and sometimes they do the damage on a driving range. Hitting 50 to 100 balls at a driving range by twisting in one direction can induce muscle spasm and pain in the low back, especially if you're tense to start with.

I saw a typical golf case recently. Lou S. was a Wall Street broker in his early forties, married, and living in a Connecticut suburb. His life was a constant rush, from the minute he got up in the morning to catch the train to Manhattan. He didn't do any exercise except play golf, and his muscles were very tight. His tension wasn't diminished on days when the train was late. It wasn't helped either by his trip downtown on the subway after the train eventually reached Grand Central. His job was demanding and full of pressures, and all day long the tension built. He left the office only to go home. By the time he arrived, he was a bundle of tension, a situation only aggravated when his wife started to tell him about the crises of her day and what the children did wrong. This hectic routine was the same from Monday through Friday. On Saturdays he got his chance to "relax" by playing golf.

One Friday evening after dinner, Mr. S. decided to go to a driving range. He had a golf game the next day, and he thought he would get ready by hitting a bucket of balls. He'd reach over, set a ball up on the tee, and whack it out. After he had done this about a dozen times, he felt a twinge in his lower back. He rubbed it briefly with his hand and then bent over to pick up another ball. This time he felt a sharp stab of pain across the lower back. As he later told me, "It was as though someone had stuck a knife into my spine." He dropped his club and sat down, but the pain was so unbearable that he rolled over on his side. Several patrons of the driving range ran to help. They thought he was having a heart attack. The pain kept up as the muscle continued in spasm. There was no way he could drive back home. In fact, there was no way he could even ride in a car. His wife was called, and after she arrived she phoned the local ambulance corps. Laid out on a stretcher, Mr. S. went home by ambulance and stayed in bed until Tuesday. On Wednesday he called me, and he came in for a visit two days later.

I took his case history and examined him. I could have gone to the files and picked out dozens of histories similar to his. I relieved the spasm with ethyl chloride spray and gentle limbering movements. When he returned a week later, I found two triggerpoints. He came back to have the triggerpoints injected, the first one on Monday, the second on Wednesday. During this period, he was not to sit for more than thirty minutes, stand for more than five minutes, or walk more than two or three blocks at a time, and as a result, he stayed at a hotel near the clinic for a week. After that he came to see me three times a week for the next three months while I gave his back muscles electrotherapy and taught him therapeutic exercises. His therapeutic exercises were similar to the relaxation, limbering, and stretching exercises in chapter 10.

Mr. S. was discharged after the three months. It's impossible to keep him away from his Saturday golf game, but he does his therapeutic exercises every day to relieve tension and keep his muscles flexible. So far, there has been no recurrence of pain.

There is one other injury to watch for in golf, and that is golf elbow. It is very similar to tennis elbow, and is caused by straining the forearm muscles to grip the club. As with tennis elbow, any triggerpoints have to be eliminated. The patient is then told to consult with the club professional for instruction on the correct grip. In a prolonged case, a golfer may also experience pain in the shoulder caused by strain or triggerpoints in the infraspinatus muscle in the shoulder.

GYMNASTICS

Anyone who does gymnastics has to be in excellent physical condition. Since every muscle in the body is used, strength and flexibility are of critical importance. Of course, certain risks are inherent in the very nature of the sport, but

the chief danger is attempting advanced feats before master-
ing the fundamentals.

A competent coach is an obvious necessity. The coach
should make sure that all the gymnasts are properly warmed
up and properly spotted. This is important for floor as well
as apparatus work. I remember one gymnastics school where
the coach required the gymnasts to warm up for twenty minutes before starting work. The coach locked the door as soon
as the warm-up started, and no latecomer was allowed to
perform.

One absolutely unnecessary danger is the trampoline. I
agree with the American Academy of Pediatrics, which several years ago recommended that trampolines be banned
from competitive sport and from physical-education programs in schools and colleges. In a three-year survey of high
school and college sports programs, the academy found that
trampolining was responsible for nine cases of permanent
paralysis and twenty-five cases of temporary paralysis. Con-
trary to popular misconception, the greatest danger comes
not from striking the edge of the trampoline but from land-
ing in the center of the mat with the cervical spine in acute
flexion. I remember the case of a nineteen-year-old boy who
was a member of a college gymnastics team. While practic-
ing on the trampoline, he performed an elementary back
drop and landed on his shoulders and back. He immediately
became numb and paralyzed in his arms and legs. Examination revealed that he had dislocated a vertebra in the spinal
cord, and he died two weeks later.

ICE SKATING

Speed skating can give you an excellent cardiovascular
workout. In our experience, skating injuries do not occur as
often as you might think. Since the ice is slippery, a fall
usually results in a sliding rather than a dead impact. It is

important that the beginner or young skater have strong support around the ankles. I have seen youngsters skate on the insides of their feet rather than on the blades, and this can cause ankle problems. Such youngsters should wear double-runner training skates. No matter what the age of the skater, the skating shoe should fit properly. Several years ago, a well-known figure skater, a young woman in her twenties, came to see me. She was in near despair. Three months previously, she had suffered pain in her right Achilles tendon. She consulted her physician, and he put her leg in a plaster cast for a month. When she resumed skating, she again had pain in the tendon and felt weaker besides. I examined her and took her case history. It turned out that her problem, as serious as it was for her, was simple to solve. The pain had started when she switched to new skating shoes. She liked them because they gave a very firm grip on the heel, but the right skate shoe was cut so that it exerted pressure on the Achilles tendon. At my suggestion, she bought new skating shoes, and the condition never recurred.

MOUNTAINEERING

Mountaineering combines strenuous physical exertion with enjoyment of the outdoors. It teaches you a respect for nature, an element missing in the lives of many people. For its enthusiasts, mountaineering fulfills a spiritual hunger to return to the very forces that have molded the earth.

There are different types of mountaineering. There is mountain hiking up relatively easy paths; higher climbing over rock, snow, and ice, where knowledge of certain techniques is essential; and the climbing of steep rock or ice, in which the climbs are numerically graded as to difficulty. In recent years, rock and ice climbing have grown tremendously in popularity, techniques have become more sophisticated, and a number of teen-agers are ascending routes that would have seemed impossible to a veteran twenty years ago.

If you are interested in mountaineering, you obviously have to be in excellent muscular and cardiovascular condition. Don't go out on your own, but accompany a knowledgeable and experienced friend or group. They are familiar with the necessary preparations and required equipment and with the various hazards encountered in every phase of this engrossing activity. Too many would-be climbers set out on their own and succumb to avoidable accidents.

Climbers, experienced climbers, do have falls, and of course there is no predicting what kind of injury a fall will inflict. I once fell sixty feet off a cliff and was saved from death only by the rope that left me dangling a few feet above a ledge. I suffered lacerations of the head, contusions of the shoulder, painful back muscles, and a very severe ankle sprain. I treated my ankle with ethyl chloride spray and immediate mobilization, I did reconditioning exercises for my back, and after the hematoma on the back was drained, I was climbing again in a few weeks.

Some climbers who use small cracks and crevices twist their fingers so repeatedly that their knuckles swell and eventually become arthritic. One leading climber who was in his late thirties came to see me and complained that he was getting dizzy when he climbed. I examined him and found a triggerpoint in the front of his neck. I eliminated it, and the dizziness went away. The state of the neck muscles is fed back to the balance centers in the brain, and the misinformation produced by the triggerpoint caused the dizziness. The climber had developed the triggerpoint from the constant strain of looking up on a particularly long and demanding climb.

SWIMMING AND DIVING

Swimming strengthens the arm and leg muscles, but not the abdominals. Moreover, different strokes produce different results. The crawl, which does not require full range of the arms, will not make the arm muscles flexible, but the breaststroke will. The crawl can also aggravate stiff necks, shoulders, or back muscles. The backstroke is permissible for a swimmer with a stiff neck or painful back muscles, but it can be difficult for anyone who has a problem extending the shoulder. The backstroke is a good general conditioner for anyone who has undergone prolonged bed rest. The butterfly should be done only by a person in excellent condition. Swimming is often recommended for the overweight because of the buoyancy of the water, and it is also a good activity for asthmatics because it promotes proper breathing.

If diving is not done under proper conditions, it can obviously lead to serious injury, including quadriplegia. High diving can cause neck injuries if the entry is not straight and back strains if the diver loses control of position on the way down.

WATER-SKIING

The leg and shoulder muscles may become too tense, especially in a beginner. Veteran or novice, the water-skier should do relaxing and stretching exercises and make sure that the legs, back, and abdominal muscles are strong as well as flexible.

FISHING

Fishermen, particularly fly-fishermen, can develop tennis elbow or shoulder strain from repetitive casting. You should be relaxed, not rigid, when you cast. If you force it or labor, improve your style by going to a casting clinic. Fishermen should also be wary of standing or sitting in the same position for more than twenty minutes at a stretch. The muscles tend to stiffen up, especially if the fisherman is wading in cold water. Deep-sea fishing for marlin, tuna, and other big fish puts a tremendous strain on the back and upper extremities, and a fisherman would be wise to do the appropriate exercises.

ROWING AND CANOEING

Canoeing and rowing can cause shoulder and back muscle strain. Like the deep-sea fisherman, the canoeist or oarsman should do appropriate exercises.

SAILING

An unusual number of sailors suffer from bad backs. They sit most of the time, and then they suddenly have to act quickly. Others hurt their back lifting a very heavy anchor.

HORSEBACK RIDING

Horseback riding requires strong leg and abdominal muscles. To strengthen the adductors on the inside of the thigh, put two fists or an object between your knees and press for ten seconds. Repeat this frequently during the day. Also do exercises for the knee and hip, plus abdominal strengthening exercises. Strong biceps muscles are required to control a frisky mount, and if these muscles need strengthening, do the weight-training exercises for the upper extremities. Neck and shoulder injuries are often suffered by those thrown from a horse, and I always advise a rider to do some gymnastics to learn how to fall.

WEIGHT LIFTING

Weight lifting builds strong muscles, but unless you take care, the muscles may lack flexibility. The injuries most common to lifters are those of the back, shoulders, and knees. These occur because the lifter lifts for strength without compensatory relaxation of the muscles. Relaxing, limbering, and stretching exercises are absolutely essential to help prevent injury. These should be done both before and after lifting.

I know a weight lifter, shot-putter and hammer-thrower named Randy. The first time I saw him work out, he obviously had very stiff muscles. He could barely reach his knees when I asked him to do the floor-touch test. I warned him he was heading for trouble, and sure enough he strained his back. I treated him, and he now follows a regular exercise program. He is more flexible than he was before, but he still is not as flexible as he should be, and he'll probably suffer another strain.

Lifting on machines, such as the Nautilus and the Universal, has the advantage of making spotting unnecessary when you lift heavy weights.

BOXING

Boxing is a first-rate sport. I am not talking about professional boxing, but boxing as conducted under Olympic rules in which a premium is placed on ring generalship. The training is demanding: running, skipping rope, and punching the light and heavy bags. The most frequent injuries are fractures of the long bones of the hand, which are likely to occur if the hands are not properly bandaged. The bags should never be punched unless the hands are bandaged. Supervised sparring or bouts should take place only between competitors of equal weight and experience. As a sport, boxing offers excellent tension release.

FENCING

Like boxing, fencing is an excellent tension releaser, but unlike boxing, fencing is unilateral. You use only one side of your body, and thus do not get an even workout. A right-handed fencer can develop a strain on the inner side of the left knee because it is used against the normal movement axis of the knee joint. Strains of the adductor muscles on the inside of the thigh and the medial collateral ligament in the knee may occur. In fencing or any other unilateral activity, it is critically important to do limbering and stretching exercises for the entire body.

JUDO, KARATE, AND WRESTLING

In judo, you are only beaten when you admit it. If you want to play macho, a joint can give, and injuries can range from dislocations to fractures. There isn't anything you can do in the way of exercise to prevent injury in judo if you don't give up in time. Warm-up and stretching exercises are essential for practice of judo throws without combat. In karate, you can strain your legs with high kicks if you are not warmed up. Back and shoulder strains occur in wrestlers who have not done sufficient stretching. To gain strength, many wrestlers also lift weights. If they do so without relaxing, limbering, and stretching their muscles, they are only adding to the potential problem.

TEAM SPORTS

I have serious reservations about some team sports and believe that, on the whole, amateurs should play them in school and not afterwards. Even then, I am definitely opposed to the concept that has made team sports the focus of physical education in our schools. In this country, where many persons are underexercised and/or overstressed, physical education in schools should be directed toward training in muscle relaxation, strengthening and stretching exercises, and building up the cardiovascular system with programs in running, cycling, swimming, hiking, tennis and fencing, and similar carry-over sports. These are sports and activities you can do as long as you live. Supplemented with an exercise program, they will keep you fit.

This is not the case with team sports, which have little value except for the athlete who plans to become a professional. If you play tennis, it's easy to find someone to play with after you're out of school, but if you're a former left tackle it's difficult to find a team. Sure, there are pickup games in the park and even office softball and touch football teams, but they're the source of many injuries. Then, as you get older, there is an increasing fitness and age gap between players, and this unduly exposes you to injury. We even see this with fathers who incur muscle strain or back pain simply while trying to teach their children the finer points of baseball or football.

FOOTBALL

Of all the team sports, football is the most conducive to injury. Even if all the players are in the same age group, football is not a contest between equals. Linemen weighing 200, 250, or 275 pounds can pile on a running back weighing only 150, or a hard-charging linebacker can spear a receiver or a quarterback with his helmet. As Dr. James Garrick, formerly of the University of Washington Sports Medicine Department, told a *New York Times* survey, "If the United States ignored an annual epidemic striking a million and a half youngsters each autumn, Americans would revolt. Yet they cheered while that many college, high school, Pop Warner, and sandlot players were injured." And Dr. Garrick added, "More high school kids get injured every Friday night than pros do in a year." In an excellent three-part series, "Brutality, the Crisis in Football," that appeared in *Sports Illustrated*, writer John Underwood noted that by mid-October of 1977, the football team at LaPorte High School in Indiana had lost fifteen lettermen because of major injuries. These included four broken backs, four broken legs, and numerous torn ligaments and cartilages. LaPorte may seem an extreme example, but in the course of a typical National Football League season, the injury rate runs at more than 100 percent. (This means a person is often injured more than once per season.) There is nothing you can do to prevent injury in football, and injury can result in permanent disability. Indeed, we have rarely seen anyone who played football in high school or college who hadn't suffered from a knee or shoulder problem.

I am not opposed to football because I am against danger in sport. If I were, I would not have been an enthusiastic motorcyclist, skier, and mountaineer. But these activities do not aim at producing injuries, and we use precaution to avoid the dangers that do exist. Without taking the challenge from the sport, football should change the rules to avoid needless injury. Teddy Roosevelt did this in 1905, and it is time it was done again. If football is tough on youngsters who are supposedly in prime physical condition, imagine what touch football is like when it's played by people who vary in age from twenty to fifty-five, most of whom are way out of shape. You don't have to be tackled to get hurt. Besides, there's nothing like a touch game between your neighbors or fellow workers to bring out old grudges. Aside from the risk of injury, which is very high, there is one other point to remember about football, tackle or touch. Although the game requires great fitness, it does not help you develop it. One game of football, even if you play every minute on offense or defense, does not do for your body what an hour of jogging will do.

I want to stress one more fact about football. It may be acceptable to professional football players to play with an injury or return to play soon after suffering one. As a physician I don't like this, but the pro players are willing to put up with this because they're getting paid, and after they make a lot of money they can retire. But this should not be allowed for the average high school and college player. Exposing him to repeated injury, just for temporary glory, is absolute folly.

SOCCER

As a physical conditioner, soccer is a much better sport than football. Soccer calls for a great deal of physical activity, especially running, and it lacks the violence of football. Nowadays a number of high schools and prep schools are switching to soccer. Not only are the costs far less than fielding a football team—a consideration in this day of tighter school budgets—but the injuries are fewer. Moreover, soccer injuries are almost never as severe as they can be in football. Soccer players sometimes suffer knee injuries, but back or shoulder injuries are relatively rare.

ICE HOCKEY

Ice hockey is a fine game, if properly played. Unfortunately, violence has become routine in the National Hockey

League, and too many youngsters are starting to follow this bad example.

BASKETBALL

Like soccer, basketball is a good conditioner, but you should be in shape when you play it. In fact, I have heard coaches say that of all team athletes, basketball players are the best conditioned. The one drawback to the game is the premium it puts on height. The shorter player doesn't stand much of a chance, which is not the case in soccer. Indeed, over the years basketball players appear to be getting taller and taller. We are now seeing more and more finger injuries that come from stuffing the ball in the basket. It's too bad that basketball isn't divided into height divisions in the same way that boxing, wrestling, and weight lifting are divided into weight classes.

BASEBALL

Although baseball is the national game, it is a very odd sport. Its physical demands are not consistent. Except for the pitcher and the catcher, most of the players stand around waiting for something to happen. Suddenly the ball is hit. The infielder or outfielder involved has to react quickly to field the ball, then throw it to home plate, second base, first base, or wherever. Coming after a period of inactivity, this sudden burst of action can bring on injury. The same applies to the base runner who has to take off at the crack of the bat.

The pitcher and the catcher are the only two players who are active all the time—but only when they are out on the field. In throwing a ball, both the pitcher and the catcher have to repeat the same movement, and as a result pitchers often end up with sore arms and shoulders. The same holds true for catchers, though to a lesser degree, because they don't have to throw the ball with the force that a pitcher does. The sore arms and shoulders are most frequently caused by muscle strain, and triggerpoints can develop just as in tennis elbow or tennis shoulder. In many cases the ailment may be misdiagnosed as "tendonitis" or some other affliction, and heat and rest prescribed. Since this does nothing to eliminate the triggerpoints, the condition does not improve. Eliminating the triggerpoints is essential. Even then the condition may recur if the player goes back to the same motion that caused the muscle strain and triggerpoints in the first place. Repeated faulty motion is the root cause of many athletic injuries.

PART TWO

Treatment and
Rehabilitation

Introduction
to
Part Two

If you suffer acute injury, you should be examined by a physician as soon as possible. After examination and treatment, you can start (with your physician's permission) to do the pertinent exercises in the following chapters to restore full strength and flexibility to the strained or sprained part.

Until you are free of pain, ethyl chloride spray or ice massage should be used to facilitate movement. Remember that movement is essential to the healing process. Do not push yourself beyond the limits of pain. Do not tire yourself. Each numbered exercise should be done three times before you move on to the next exercise. Always be sure to complete the exercises by repeating them in reverse order so that you end with the exercise with which you began.

In acute cases, do just the first few exercises, but do them several times a day if you can. As pain subsides, add exercises, but again, try to do them several times a day. Later, when your pain has subsided and you have begun to work on strengthening your muscles, you may increase repetition of movements. Reduce the number of sessions gradually to two, then finally one a day.

Note: If you suffer an injury to a lower extremity, do not walk without crutches until you can do so without limping or suffering pain.

6

A New Treatment:
Movement and
Ethyl Chloride

It used to be that when patients came to see me after suffering an injury, they would ask, "Can I play again?" Now they usually ask, *"When* can I play again?"

When a person suffers an injury, most physicians will recommend the RICE treatment. RICE stands for rest, ice, compression, and elevation. Instead of RICE, I use the MECE treatment for many injuries. MECE stands for movement, ethyl chloride, and elevation. Rest does not promote healing, whereas movement does.

MECE

Many years ago, as a resident in surgery at the University of Vienna Hospital, I was in the emergency fracture service. We took care of fractures, sprains (partial tears of a ligament), and strains (partial tears of a muscle). We routinely treated all acute sprains and strains by immobilizing the patients. In a mild case, we used a soft bandage, while in more severe cases we would immobilize the patients with splints or plaster casts. When someone suffered a severe sprain of the knee, we would encase the knee in a long plaster cylinder. Had it not been for an old friend, Heinz Kowalski, I undoubtedly would have continued with the old methods of treatment. Kowalski was an athletic coach and gym owner who came from a family of circus acrobats. He was very highly regarded as a coach. In fact, he was then president of the Austrian Sports Teachers Association. One day after I finished working out at his gym, we fell to talking. Kowalski had sent a number of patients to the university hospital, but he had never sent anyone with a strain or sprain, and I asked him why.

"Because you doctors don't know how to treat a sprain or a strain," he said.

"What do you mean?" I asked. "We know what we're doing."

"No, you don't," Kowalski said. "You immobilize anyone with a sprain or strain by wrapping them in bandages or plaster casts."

"You have to do that to heal the injury," I retorted.

"That's your way, not mine," he said. "In the circus we had to perform. If we sprained a wrist or strained a muscle and we immobilized the injury the way you do, we wouldn't be able to perform. If we couldn't perform, we didn't eat, so we didn't immobilize our injuries. I'd take a cloth or a towel, soak it in alcohol, wrap it around the injured part and then expose the towel to hot steam. That produced numbness in the part, and I could start to move it. I'd do this several times during the day, and after a day or two, I was usually ready to perform again."

I was intrigued by what Kowalski had to say, and I decided to check on his method. My chance came a few days later when two men arrived at the hospital with sprained ankles which they had hurt skiing. While I was examining them, one of them said they weren't looking forward to a month of wearing plaster casts on their legs, because they both wanted to get back to skiing as soon as possible. I told them about my conversation with Kowalski and asked if they wanted to try his method. There was no guarantee it would work, but then again it might. If it didn't work, we would know soon enough and put on the casts. They said they wanted to try Kowalski's method. They did, and in only three days they had full use of their ankles.

I then began to experiment with other fluids that might be more effective than alcohol compresses, such as mixtures of ether, acetone, and other chemicals. I tried ethyl chloride, which we sometimes used as a general anesthetic but mainly as a local anesthetic when making small incisions and lancing boils. Ethyl chloride produces a local anesthesia by cooling the skin. It seemed promising to me. The first patient I treated with it was a veterinarian who came limping in on two canes with a severely sprained ankle. The pain, he said, was excruciating. I sprayed ethyl chloride on the ankle, and I then had him move it up and down and in and out. The pain ebbed. I sprayed the ankle again and had him exercise the ankle until he said he felt reasonably comfortable. He came back to the hospital three times that week for additional treatments. After the third visit, he said his ankle was all right. I asked him to come back in a month for a checkup. Meanwhile, he was to inform me immediately if there was any difficulty with the ankle. A month later the vet came back for his checkup. His ankle was in fine shape, and after I finished examining him, he smiled and said, "You've got a good thing with that ethyl chloride spray."

"What exactly do you mean by that?" I asked.

"I've started using it in my practice on horses and dogs," he said. "I shave the sprained leg and spray it with ethyl chloride. It works exceptionally well. Almost all the animals run off after treatment."

Afterwards, I began treating all my hospital patients with ethyl chloride spray. It works on any strain or sprain because it relieves muscle spasm. This allows the patient to begin to move, and movement helps relieve swelling. As I used the spray on more and more patients, I learned empirically that immobilization was not necessary for healing.

I checked the records of patients with wrist fractures who wore plaster casts from the wrist to above the elbow. Some did no exercise at all, while others flexed and extended their fingers, moved their shoulder up and down, and put their hand behind their neck and back. These exercises kept the muscles active and improved circulation to the whole extremity. My review revealed that the patients who made the quickest and the best recoveries were those who had exercised the most, even if they had suffered worse fractures than patients who hadn't exercised. As a result, the hospital started a special department to give exercises to all fracture patients. The effects were so beneficial that the hospital then gave all trauma patients special exercises to reestablish their muscular strength and flexibility. Although most physicians nowadays are aware that exercise has a key role to play in rehabilitation, few know how and when to prescribe the appropriate exercises for a given injury.

When I gave a paper on the use of ethyl chloride spray to the Academy of Physicians in Vienna, a correspondent for the American Medical Association who attended the meeting sent an abstract to the *Journal* of the AMA, which published it in 1935. I began teaching a course in the use of ethyl chloride spray at the Vienna Medical School, where a number of American physicians became my students.

Around this time, a French neurosurgeon wrote a paper in which he theorized that a sprain is primarily an irritation of the sympathetic nervous system and that an injection of procaine would give immediate relief. It's true that an injection of procaine in an acute sprain or strain will relieve pain and that if you keep the part moving you will get over the acute phase. But this practice presents two great dangers, which is why we don't use procaine injections in treatment of an acute injury. First of all, procaine can eliminate the pain in a major injury, and the last thing you want to do with a major ligament tear or a major fracture is to move it. Obviously you can't treat a major ligament tear with ethyl chloride spray, but you don't have to worry about using ethyl chloride because it is self-limiting. It will relieve pain from strains and sprains but not from major ligament tears or major fractures. Ethyl chloride will work for fractures that do not require immobilization because they are minor and do not cause any displacement. The other drawback to the use of procaine is rebound effect. A patient injected with procaine might be back with more pain the next day. Why? Because the patient reinjured the numbed part while under the influence of the procaine and became much worse off.

I remember one dramatic case that illustrates the differences between using ethyl chloride spray and injecting procaine into an injury. When I was working as a fracture surgeon at the College of Physicians and Surgeons at Columbia University, a colleague of mine brought a twelve-year-old boy to see me. The boy, who was the son of another physician, had returned from horseback riding complaining of a stiff and painful neck. Since he hadn't been thrown from the horse, no X ray had been taken. My colleague said to me, "Let's see you work your miracle with ethyl chloride spray." I sprayed the boy's neck, but he still complained of the pain. An X ray was ordered immediately. It showed a compression fracture of the third cervical vertebra, which was tuberculous. The youngster had a broken neck. Had I injected procaine to kill the pain, he probably would have become a quadriplegic when he moved his neck.

In our clinic, we regularly use ethyl chloride spray for the treatment of strains and sprains. Let's say you're a jogger who has a sprained knee. I first find out where your pain is most severe. If the pain is most severe in the medial collateral ligament of the knee, I spray the area with ethyl chloride and then have you bend and extend the knee two or three times. If you still have pain, I'll ask you to show me where. The pain usually shifts from the more acutely damaged area to a less damaged area because limitation of motion has concealed it until now. The idea is to follow the pain with the spray. I spray this area and have you bend and extend the knee two or three times, rest briefly, then move the knee again. If there is no pain, you may walk out of the clinic. A minor sprain will respond to ethyl chloride spray and gentle exercise of the affected part with immediate recovery. However, if a sprain of the lower extremities is more severe, you must use crutches until you can walk normally without pain or limping. If you walk before that, you will stiffen the affected part of the leg or knee and walk as though the leg were a stick. Then the entire leg will stiffen up and your problem will only get worse.

USING ETHYL CHLORIDE SPRAY

Ordinarily, ethyl chloride is used only by a physician, but the doctor may prescribe it. Here are the correct procedures to follow when using ethyl chloride spray and movement in treatment of an injury. *Note:* Avoid using ethyl chloride spray or storing it near an open flame; it is flammable. Avoid inhalation; it is a general anesthetic. Because of these qualities, several people advocate the use of other coolant sprays, but I do not find them nearly as effective as ethyl chloride.

The painful region must be determined through gentle movement by the patient. The movement must be in the direction in which motion is impaired. Movement should never be brusque or abrupt. This is especially important in treating muscle spasm.

The ethyl chloride is then sprayed on the painful area with the nozzle held three to eight inches from the skin. Excessive spraying can cause frostbite.

The patient then starts gentle movement of the part involved, again in the direction in which motion has been painful and limited. As the patient carefully increases move-

ment, new painful areas—concealed until now through the
limitation of motion—will develop. These areas, too, have to
be sprayed, and movement must be resumed after each spray
application.

A treatment should last between ten and thirty minutes. It
should be conducted with care and within the limits of pain.

A single treatment will take care of mild strains or sprains,
but patients with more severe strains or sprains will need
treatment every day during the first week and every other
day later on. Effective treatment of the injury should not
require the use of ethyl chloride spray after the second
week.

Common mistakes made in treating a patient with ethyl
chloride spray and exercise are:

failure to cover the entire painful area with spray.
having the patient do violent exercise.
neglect of the patient's pain limit.
failure by the patient to exercise the injured part at home.
prolonged and excessive use of an injured part, such as
    walking or standing on a weak or painful leg.
failure to have follow-up treatments.

You may wonder why ethyl chloride spray, a surface anesthetic, has deep beneficial effect. One theory is that pain,
originating in one point of the sensory motor chain, leads to
reflex muscle spasm and locking of joints. The sensory motor
chain consists of sensory receptor, reflex center, motor nerve,
muscle, and nerve. Pain originating in the sensory portion of
the reflex is either in the joint or muscle and leads to muscle
spasm. Elimination of the pain at any point in the chain
breaks the chain and causes relaxation of the muscle spasm.
We don't know exactly how ethyl chloride spray breaks the
chain, but the important thing is, it does. However, it is also
important to remember that ethyl chloride spray alone, without movement, will not achieve satisfactory results.

7

*Other Treatments
for Injury*

There are other modes of treatment that can be used in case of injury. However, it is important to know what should be used, when, and how.

ICE

You may have heard that ice will help strains and sprains. Although not as effective as ethyl chloride spray, ice can be used. Don't apply an ice pack, however, because it limits movement. Instead perform ice massage. How do you go about it? Fill a paper cup with water and put it in the freezer. When it is frozen, take it out and remove the rim. You now have a cup of ice you can hold comfortably in your hand while you rub the ice back and forth over the injured area. If you're in a hurry, use an ice cube and a glove. After you have gone back and forth over the injured area, start movement. If you have hurt your ankle, start moving it up and down. When that movement is less painful, move the ankle in and out. Then start flexing and extending your toes.

If you have hurt your knee, bend and extend it, then rub ice over the area to lessen the pain. You can use ice massage for any other joint or muscle area that you want to treat.

HEAT

Never use heat or hot packs for sprains or strains of the upper and lower extremities. Heat will increase swelling and bleeding from the capillary blood vessels. However, heat can be used to treat a muscle spasm in the low back. The procedure is simple. Lie on your stomach and have a helper soak a towel in very hot water. The helper should wring out the towel completely and place it on your back. The towel will cool quickly, so repeated applications should be made for fifteen minutes. After that, start doing back-pain exercises 1 through 4 in chapter 10 while your helper ice-massages the spasm area or sprays it with ethyl chloride.

Infrared heat, which has a soothing effect on muscles, can be helpful before massage and exercise. Deep heat, short-wave diathermy, should never be used for acute injuries, although it may be useful in treatment of old chronic muscle or joint pain. I do not recommend a whirlpool bath for the treatment of sprains and strains because it restricts movement and is not effective. Instead, take a good strong shower, alternating hot (but not too hot) and cold water. A hot bath can be relaxing, but most tubs today are so small they do not allow complete relaxation of the body.

ELECTROTHERAPY

In treating a patient with an injured muscle, I often use an electric current (sinusoidal wave) that makes the muscle contract rhythmically. This helps to strengthen the muscle and to warm it for future exercise. In the case of acute back and neck muscle strains, before the sinusoidal current I use a tetanizing current, which causes a strong contraction of

82 HANS KRAUS, M.D.

the muscle. This fatigues the muscle so that it relaxes when the current is discontinued.

MASSAGE

A good massage is wonderfully relaxing for the muscles, but unfortunately massage is becoming a lost art. Few physical therapists or masseurs today know how to give a good one. Too many give massages that can be harmful.

Massage can be a useful aid in rehabilitating an injury. However, it should be given only under a physician's direction because it might otherwise worsen the injury. Massage is also useful in relaxing muscles before sports and in relieving fatigue and soreness afterwards.

Some basic techniques must be kept in mind. The masseur should use talcum powder rather than oil because oil makes kneading difficult. A massage should always "flow with the lymphs" by beginning at the end of the extremity and moving up. In massaging a leg, for example, the masseur should begin with the toes and then do the sole and sides of the feet and the heel before moving up the leg. Back massage should begin at the lower back and move up. Similarly, neck massage should begin at the base of the neck.

A massage can cover the whole body or localized areas. A good massage is divided into two parts requiring two different techniques, one following the other. First the masseur uses the technique known as effleurage. Here the masseur places one hand over the other and strokes the painful area with a circular motion as though polishing a table. After effleuraging the back, legs, arms, or neck, the masseur then employs the kneading massage technique on the muscles. Here the masseur lightly but firmly grasps the muscles between the fingers and thumbs of both hands. The fingers then alternately knead them in a rolling, rhythmic fashion. After exertion, kneading massage helps to prevent development of a charley horse.

If a muscle is sore, the masseur can also help to alleviate the soreness by using a third technique, deep-point massage. The masseur puts two fingers of one hand together and holds them in place with the other hand. The masseur then presses on the sore muscle area and gently rotates the two fingers. Tight and tender muscles can benefit from deep-point massage.

Some observations about massage: If you're right-handed, you or the masseur may notice that the muscles on your left side are tighter than those on the right. This is because you use the right arm to reach while you use the left hand for holding. The opposite condition may hold true if you are left-handed.

Avoid massage entirely if you have phlebitis or varicose veins. With phlebitis, massage will irritate the veins, and if the veins are thrombosed (i.e., closed), blood clots may be dislodged.

Always avoid rough massages, such as triggerpoint massage, in which the masseur attempts to crush a triggerpoint with the knuckles or a rod. It is still practiced occasionally, but triggerpoints should be eliminated not by crushing but by needling and injection as I noted previously. Also avoid "hacking" massage in which the masseur's hands and fingers chop at a muscle.

In recent years, a Japanese massage technique known as shiatsu has come into vogue. In shiatsu, the masseur places pressures on the so-called acupuncture points, and the massage is sometimes known as "acupressure." Although shiatsu can be helpful, it should only be given by an expert, and unfortunately there are few around.

Some persons suffer from a condition known as fibrositis. Although this condition causes no limitation of motion, to the person suffering from it the skin feels thicker, is exquisitely tender, and aches. Fibrositis occurs on the shoulders and the upper and lower back. Women may also develop it on the seat or the sides of the legs. Specialists in physical medicine have known of the condition for a long time. A year ago, however, the French popular press discovered fibrositis, and all sorts of alleged remedies for it have been described in books now translated into English. Be wary; more must be learned about this condition. In our experience, relief can only be obtained—and then not always—from a rolling or pinching massage. But again, remember, the massage must be performed by an expert under the direction of a knowledgeable physician.

SELF-HYPNOSIS

Self-hypnosis is an excellent way to attain deep relaxation and relief from tension or pain within minutes. The American Medical Association has accepted hypnosis as a legitimate modality of treatment. I have found it very useful in patients who are highly hypnotizable. Transcendental meditation is used by many people, but TM cannot be used at a moment's notice as self-hypnosis can. You can learn self-hypnosis from a competent physician, psychiatrist, or psychologist.

Several years ago, a young woman who had been training for the U.S. national equestrian team came to see me with painful shoulders and a stiff neck. The cause of her problem was her coach, of whom she was very much afraid. I found triggerpoints in her shoulder girdle and neck muscles, treated them, and she returned to training. Soon she was back again with pain because she tensed up as soon as she rode for the coach. Fortunately, she was highly hypnotizable. She quickly learned how to use self-hypnosis to relax and to overcome her fear of the coach. She made the team.

DMSO

I am aware of the claims made for DMSO, but I caution the reader that its use has not been approved by the FDA.

8

Rehabilitation after Injury: The Upper Extremities

SHOULDER STRAIN OR SPRAIN AND INCOMPLETE SHOULDER SEPARATION

The shoulder joint has a very loose capsule, so before it is affected, the surrounding muscles become strained. The insertion of the muscles at the shoulder, the so-called tendinous or rotator cuff, can also be strained or suffer minor tears. Major tears may require surgery, but minor tears can be mobilized like any other sprain. Recently I saw a skier who had fallen and partially torn his rotator cuff. When surgery was suggested, he came in for a second opinion. I decided that the tear was small and put him on an exercise program using ethyl chloride spray and electrotherapy. Within three weeks he was discharged with full range and power in the shoulder, and he immediately returned to skiing and all normal activities. If this patient had undergone surgery, he would have been immobilized from four to six weeks, and then he would have needed several months of rehabilitation.

In another recent case, a cyclist sought a second opinion for a shoulder injury. He had fallen off his bike and separated the acromioclavicular joint. Scheduled for surgery, he asked for my opinion. I found the separation to be minor and put him on exercise therapy. Four weeks later he had complete use of the shoulder and full strength.

The exercises for a strained or sprained shoulder or an incomplete shoulder separation are given below. In the beginning you may be able to do only the first two or three exercises. Don't push yourself, but gradually add exercises as tolerated.

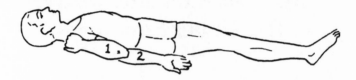

1. Make a fist, touch your shoulder with the fist, then let your forearm down and unclench the fist.

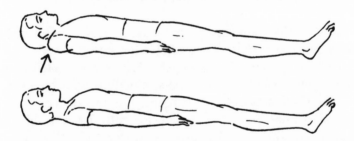

2. Shrug your shoulders and relax.

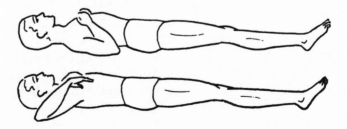

3. Lie on your back, put your hands on your chest, and move your elbows as high as you can. Return to starting position and relax.

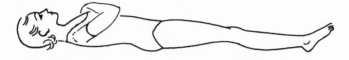

4. Reach over to the opposite side of your chest with the arm of your injured shoulder. Return to the starting position and relax.

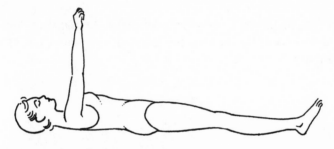

5. Reach straight up with the arm of your injured shoulder, bring it down, and relax.

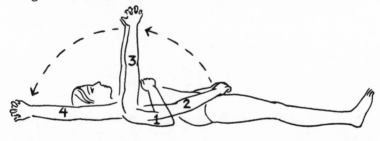

6. Join your hands over your chest and bring them down toward your legs. Now raise them slowly as far as you can and bring them back straight over your head. On the way down to the starting position, press the hand of the injured shoulder on the other hand. This will help you avoid discomfort.

The following exercises, which are more advanced, are to be done sitting or standing.

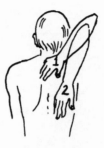

7. Touch the back of your neck with the hand of the injured shoulder, then move the hand down your back as far as you can.

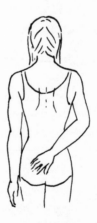

8. Touch your lower back with the hand of your injured shoulder.

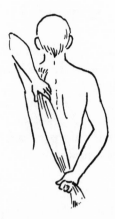

9. Take a towel with the hand of your good shoulder and put it behind your back. Now take the loose end in your other hand and pull the hand of the injured shoulder toward your neck.

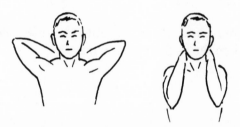

10. Fold your ams behind your neck and bring the elbows back. Bring the elbows forward, then relax. Repeat all exercises in reverse.

BURSITIS

Many so-called cases of bursitis or baseball sore shoulder are caused by triggerpoints in the shoulder muscles. After treatment for triggerpoints, do the exercises for shoulder strain and sprain.

ELBOW SPRAIN

Elbow sprain is rare, but when it occurs, patients often mistakenly attempt to stretch the elbow flexors by carrying a heavy weight in their hand. I have had patients come to me with bent arms that they could not straighten out because they had carried a bucket of water. *Do not carry a heavy weight. This will only perpetuate the flexion.*

The exercises are as follows.

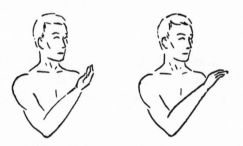

1. Put your hand to the opposite shoulder, look into the palm and then the back of your hand.

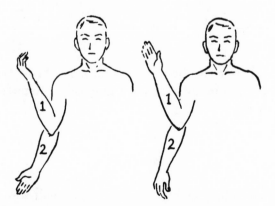

2. Bend and extend the elbow with the palm facing up and then with the palm facing down.

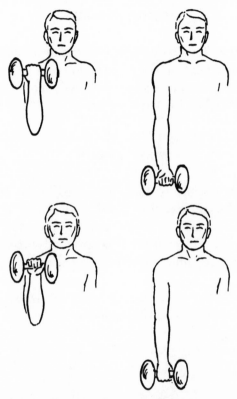

3. When the elbow feels stronger, hold a comfortable weight in your hand and bend and extend the elbow.

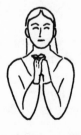 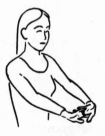

4. To stretch elbow flexors, join your hands as if in prayer, fingers interlocked, turn the hands so you see the backs, and then stretch your arms.

TENNIS ELBOW

Tennis elbow is usually caused by the development of one or more triggerpoints in the forearm muscles near the elbow. After the triggerpoints and pain are eliminated, do the exercises listed below for wrist sprain.

WRIST SPRAIN

Before you do any of these exercises, make certain that you don't have any fracture of the small bones of the wrists. The scaphoid bone close to the radius in the wristbone often breaks in a fall. To rehabilitate a sprained wrist or forearm muscles that were afflicted with tennis elbow, do the following exercises.

1. Support your arm on a table, your wrist projecting. Bring the wrist up, then bring it down.

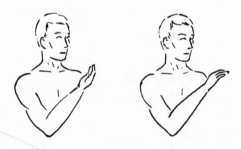

2. Put your arm on the opposite shoulder, turning the wrist out. Look into your palm and then turn your wrist to see the back of your hand.

3. Make a fist, open, and spread the fingers.

When your wrist feels stronger, you can add these exercises to the program.

4. Pick up a one-pound weight. Put your wrist over the edge of a table, bend it down, and then extend it with the weight in hand.

5. Wring out a wet towel. You can also knead putty or use a spring strengthener for the fingers.

FINGER SPRAIN AND BASEBALL FINGER

Finger sprain can be treated immediately with movement, ethyl chloride spray, and the exercises given below. However, if the tip of the finger, the last phalanx, is bent down (what we call "baseball finger"), the probable cause is a tear of the extensor tendon. This condition usually requires immobilization in hyperextension with a splint to restore full extension. After that, the exercises given here can be used to recondition the finger.

1. Bend the injured finger and extend it.

2. Spread the fingers open, then close them.

3. Make a fist, open it, and spread the fingers, first with the thumb outside, then with the thumb inside. Repeat the exercises in reverse.

9

Rehabilitation After Injury: The Lower Extremities

PULLED GROIN MUSCLE

A pulled groin muscle is a strain of the adductor muscles at the insertion of the pubic bone. It is frequently suffered by joggers and runners. It should be treated as an acute muscle strain with ethyl chloride spray and movement.

The exercises for a pulled groin muscle are:

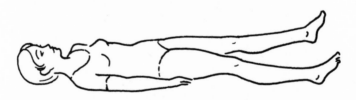

1. Lie down on your back with your legs extended and together. Spread the legs, bring them back together, and relax.

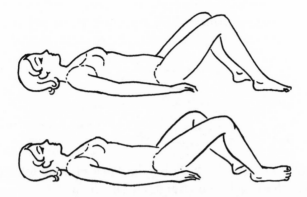

2. Do the same exercise but with the knees bent. Alternate the two exercises. In a chronic case, a physician should check for triggerpoints.

HIP STRAIN

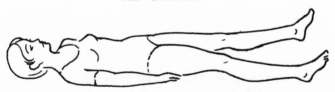

1. Lie on your back with your legs extended and together. Then spread legs apart. Return to starting position and relax.

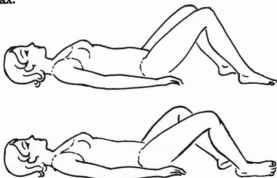

2. Lie on your back with your knees flexed and together. Spread knees as far as you can and bring them back together.

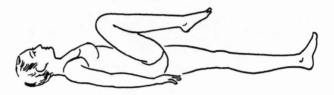

3. Still on your back, bring the knee of your injured hip to your chest and then straighten out. Relax.

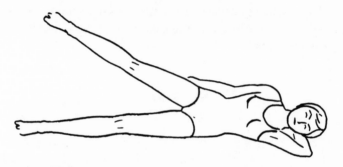

4. Lie on your good side and lift your injured leg sideways. Lower it and relax.

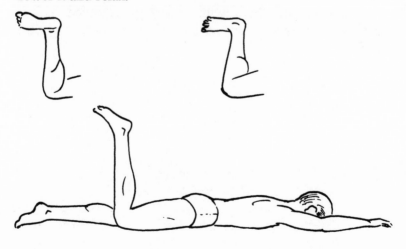

5. Lie on your stomach, bend the knee of your injured leg, and then turn the leg to one side and then the other.

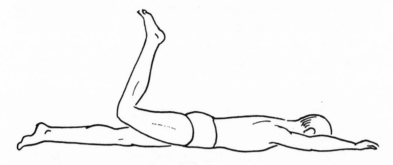

6. Still on your stomach, bend the knee of your injured leg and lift the leg as high as you can. Lower it and relax.

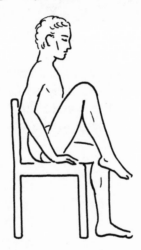

7. Sit in a chair, bring the knee of your injured leg to your chest, then relax.

CHARLEY HORSE

Charley horse is muscle fatigue. Although the condition is generally confined to the thighs, it can occur elsewhere. A mild case is best treated by doing the relaxing, limbering, and stretching exercises that pertain to the muscle in question. Kneading massage is also helpful. A severe charley horse can also be treated with ethyl chloride spray, hot packs, or hot showers. A charley horse is not an acute trauma, so do not worry that heat may cause bleeding and swelling.

PULLED HAMSTRING

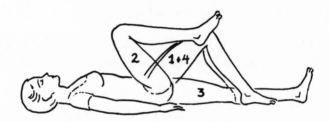

1. Lie on your back with your knees flexed. Slowly draw the knee of the injured leg as close to your chest as you comfortably can. Return the foot to the floor, slide the leg out straight, then slide it back to the knee-flexed position and relax.

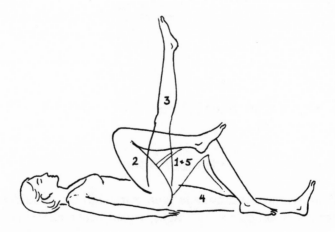

2. Lie on your back, knees flexed. Bring the knee of the injured leg as close to your chest as possible, then extend the leg straight up with the toes pointed toward the ceiling. Lower the straight leg to the floor, then slide it back to the flexed position.

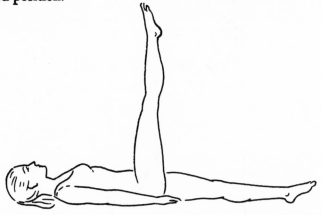

3. Lie on your back and raise the injured leg slowly as high as you can, keeping the knee straight. Lower the leg to the starting position.

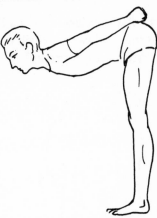

4. When the hamstring feels better, stand up, feet together, and clasp your hands behind your back. Bend over

from the hips as far as you can and raise your head until you feel stretching in the back of your legs.

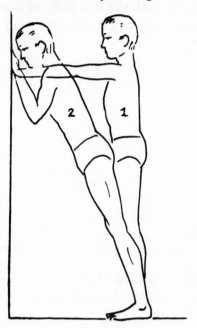

5. Place both hands flat against the wall at shoulder height. Slowly lean into the wall as far as you can go, keeping your body straight and heels on the ground. Then push back to starting position.

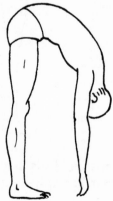

6. Stand up straight, your heels together. Relax by inhaling and exhaling deeply. Now drop your neck gradually and let your trunk hang loose from the hips. Gradually drop your shoulders and then your back. Do this easily, two or three times. When you are completely relaxed and "hanging from the hips," reach down as far as you can. Be sure to keep knees straight. Do not strain.

KNEE SPRAIN, PARTIAL TEAR OF THE LIGAMENTOUS APPARATUS OF THE KNEE JOINT

If you can't walk normally without pain or limping, you must use crutches. Moreover, if there is considerable swelling inside the knee, stay off your feet and rest as much as possible. Treat the sprain with ethyl chloride spray once or twice a day, and start to do the exercises given below. Early mobilization and exercise are essential for the healing process. Electrotherapy can also be helpful in treating the vastus medialis and the popliteal muscle in the knee.

Major tears of the ligament may require surgery. Although surgery should be avoided if possible, it can be a godsend when needed. A prime example is a tear of the meniscus of the knee joint. Today, thanks to microsurgery, the operation can be performed without exposing the knee joint. Moreover, the patient is usually able to leave the hospital within a day and start rehabilitation. As a result, there is hardly any loss of strength or flexibility. Having undergone this microsurgery myself, I can vouch that I was cross-country skiing ten days after leaving the hospital.

In nonsurgical cases of knee sprain, exercising can begin at once, while in surgical cases, exercising can begin as soon as the surgeon permits. At the start the surgeon may recommend such mild exercises as toe flexing, leg raises, and muscle tightening and relaxation.

KNEE EXERCISES

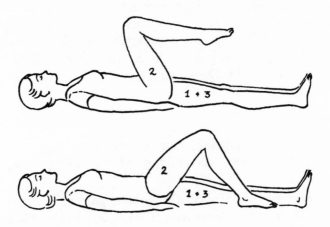

1. Lie on your back, gently bend and extend the injured knee. If this is difficult to do, don't raise the heel but slide it back and forth as far as you can.

2. Tighten the quadriceps, the muscles in the front of the thigh. If you can't do this, tighten the quads in the uninjured leg and then try to tighten the quads in both legs at the same time.

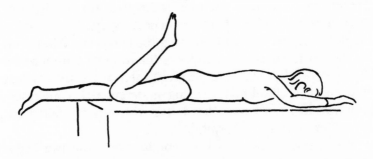

3. Lie on your stomach with your foot over the edge of a bed. Bend your knee and bring your foot as far back as you can, then extend the leg again.

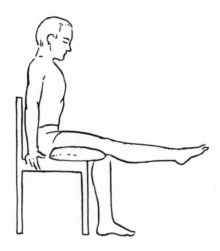

4. After you're able to do the above exercises with your knee completely straightened, you're ready to work against gravity. Sit in a chair or on a table with a pillow beneath the injured knee while the uninjured leg rests securely on the floor. Now extend the injured leg to 180 degrees. Move very slowly into this exercise. Keep in mind that you should attempt this gravity exercise only after you've been able to straighten your leg in a supported position. If you try to do this exercise before your leg is ready, you can set yourself back considerably.

Being able to hold your leg straight against gravity is a sign that you're ready to lift your leg with weights on it. Fill cloth bags with beans or shot, one pound to a bag, or buy a weight-lifting boot. Do the following weight-lifting exercise only every other day. It is important that you rest between weight-bearing sessions. Do the non-weight-bearing exercises daily.

5. Before attaching any weight, sit on the edge of a chair with a pillow under your injured knee. Turn your toes outward so the inner aspect of your knee gets more of the stress. Now slowly raise your leg until it is completely extended. Do this three times.

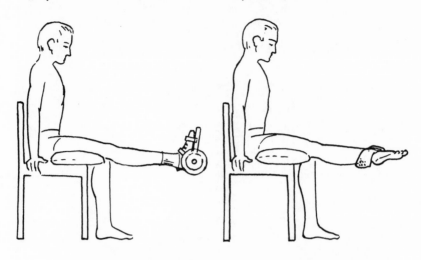

6. Sitting on the edge of a chair, place a one-pound weight over your instep and again turn your toes outward and raise your leg until it is completely extended. Lift the weight three times. If you find this easy to do, keep adding weight in one-pound increments until you feel the knee getting tired or you find it difficult to hold the leg completely extended. At this point, don't stop, but remove the weights gradually as you repeat the exercise. Finish with the five non-weight-lifting exercises in reverse order.

When your physician finally allows you to stand on your leg with your full body weight on it, you can test its strength compared with the normal leg.

1. Stand up and bend both knees. Do both bend easily?

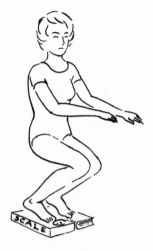

2. Take a bathroom scale and a book the same thickness as the scale. Stand with the foot of the normal leg on the scale, the other on the book. Do a knee bend and have some-one note the amount of weight shown on the scale. Now reverse the scale and the book so that the foot of the injured leg is on the scale, the other on the book. Do a knee bend and note the weight shown. Any difference in pounds is an indication of muscle weakness in the injured leg.

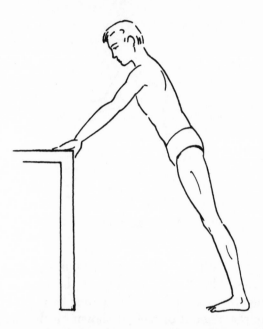

3. Measure your upper calf muscle flexibility. Hold on to the edge of a sturdy table and lean forward with both heels on the floor. Compare the good with the injured leg.

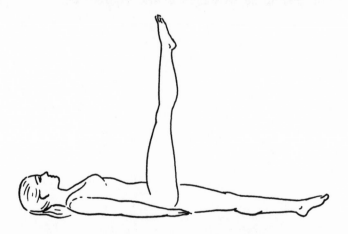

4. Measure hamstring flexibility. Lie flat on your back and

raise each leg straight up, one at a time. You should aim for an elevation of at least eighty degrees with each leg.

If your leg is able to bear weight, but you still walk with a limp or an awkward gait, your quadriceps may be weak and the knee flexors (hamstring and calf muscles) stiff and tight. In this case, continue to walk with crutches and do the following exercises.

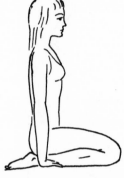

1. Get on your knees and sit back on your heels. If this is difficult, support your weight with your hands.

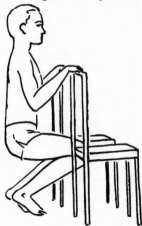

2. Stand between two chairs for support and do three knee bends.

If you have been in a short cast below the knee and were able to keep strength and tone in your thigh, you will have to concentrate on reconditioning your calf muscles. If you're not ready to do toe stands, do the following resistive exercise for the calf muscles.

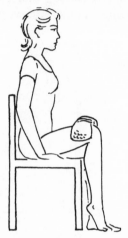

1. Sit in a chair with your foot resting flat on the floor. Lift your heel to a toe-stand position. Now put a one-pound weight on your knee to make the exercise a little harder. Keep adding weights up to tolerance.

I have devoted a number of exercises to the knee because too many people suffer needlessly from knee injuries. And too many people reinjure their knees. Given the proper exercises, this need not be the case at all, as our records show. I did a follow-up on 208 patients with ligamentous knee joint injuries that I treated with ethyl chloride spray and exercise therapy immediately after injury. Fifty-seven of these patients, it should be noted, had previously suffered injury to the same knee joint before they came to see us. Follow-up examination showed that of the 208 treated, 148 of them, 71.2 percent, had what we called good results. The injured knee was perfectly normal and equal in every way to the uninjured knee, and all 148 patients had returned to their regular sports and activities. Fifty-six patients, 26.9 percent, had what we called fair results, based on three criteria: (1) they were not able to resume all sports, or (2) the knee was slightly symptomatic (that is, it was easily fatigued or had occasional pain), or (3) the knee was less strong or less flexible than normal. If any one of these three criteria was present, we listed recovery as fair. Four patients, 1.9 percent, had what we called poor results. They failed two or more of the conditions listed above.

In another follow-up, thirty-nine of the fifty-seven patients who had previously suffered one or more injuries to the knee we reconditioned replied to our questionnaire. Thirty-three said the knee was fine. In fact, many of them said the knee was stronger than before the original injury. Six patients said they had reinjured themselves during strenuous athletic activity. Two of them had not reconditioned the knee to full strength, and we had warned two others not to participate in athletic activity until treatment had been concluded. In other words, there were only two fully reconditioned patients who suffered reinjury.

In a two- to fifteen-year follow-up of seventy skiers, many of whom had suffered more than one injury to the same knee, we found that sixty-two skied without difficulty, five had no complaints but were not interested in skiing, and only three returned to skiing with complaints of occasional pain and swelling. No one suffered reinjury.

Braces and supports have their place, but our general philosophy is that they should be used only for temporary protection. We don't let patients get "married" to them.

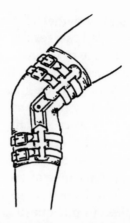

The knee brace with hinges on both sides allows a knee to bend, stretch, and extend. It protects the knee against lateral force, but is less effective against rotational motion.

When the cruciate ligaments are torn, the knee often becomes permanently unstable. Surgery is required as soon as possible after this injury. If surgery is delayed, the condition becomes more complicated, and good results are difficult to obtain. If the knee does not receive surgical attention, the derotation brace designed by Dr. James Nicholas is needed for stabilization.

CHRONIC DISLOCATION OF THE KNEECAP

If the kneecap (patella) is dislocated frequently, causing swelling and disability, surgery is necessary. Reconditioning exercises for the knee may begin as soon as the surgeon permits.

OSGOOD-SCHLATTER'S DISEASE

This is not actually a disease but a growth retardation of the knee in adolescents. Leave the knee alone and avoid sports and exercise that aggravate the pain. The patient will usually outgrow the condition in time.

SHIN SPLINTS

Shin splints can be caused by flat feet, inadequate shoes, running on a hard surface, running without a warm-up, or any combination thereof. Find the cause, or you will suffer from shin splints again.

A mild case can be treated with ethyl chloride spray or ice massage. Do the ankle-sprain exercises given below, but be sure to extend the foot to maximum extension and use ethyl chloride or ice massage while doing so.

A chronic case of shin splints may be caused by triggerpoints and should be treated accordingly. Electrotherapy can also be used to relax the muscles after treatment.

Sometimes muscles affected by shin splints can swell to the point where they compress the nerves and blood vessels in the compartment formed by the fascia in which the muscles are encased. The condition, known as anterior compartment syndrome, may require surgery. See also the entry on fatigue or stress fractures in chapter 11.

CALF-MUSCLE TEAR

A calf-muscle tear usually responds well to immediate mobilization, but not to immediate weight-bearing if the tear is severe. Inasmuch as the calf muscle is a knee and ankle muscle, knee and ankle exercises should be done to restore it to full strength and flexibility. Failure to warm up properly is often the cause of calf-muscle tear. I see a growing number of patients who suffer calf, knee, and ankle injuries because their legs cannot withstand the prolonged pounding of running on pavement. Only recently I saw an executive who, after running his third marathon, came in with pain in his calf and groin muscles that he had tried to "run out." He suffered from triggerpoints that had to be needled and injected, and he is now on a reconditioning program doing therapeutic exercise. He has given up the marathon and is going to restrict his running to three to five miles a day on resilient ground. Although I am very much opposed to giving up anything athletically, the marathon, as I noted in chapter 5, does impose stress on many people.

PLANTARIS LONGUS TEAR

The plantaris longus muscle runs from the back of the knee to the heel. When it tears, it feels as though the back of the leg had been struck with a stick or a whip, much like the sensation felt by the tear of an Achilles tendon or a calf muscle. As with calf-muscle tear, knee and ankle exercises should be performed.

ACHILLES TENDON TEAR

Tear of the Achilles tendon requires immediate surgery and immobilization. When the surgeon permits reconditioning to begin, ankle and knee exercises should be performed to restore strength and flexibility to the entire extremity.

ACHILLES TENDONITIS

True inflammation of the Achilles tendon requires rest and anti-inflammatory medication. Note that this condition is often simulated by tightness and/or triggerpoints in the soleus muscle of the calf.

ANKLE SPRAIN

Treatment within the first twenty-four or forty-eight hours after injury will relieve a mild sprain of the ankle considerably, and normal work and play may be resumed at once. In more severe cases the disability may last longer, and in very severe cases be protracted. Whatever the case, the ankle should be examined and treated as soon as possible by a physician.

Sprain of the ankle joint may affect both the upper and lower ankle joint and the joints of the foot. Acute sprains should be treated immediately with ethyl chloride spray and movement. If your ankle does not respond fully and you find it painful to walk, you must use crutches to avoid worsening the condition. If relief follows with the spray treatment and movement, there is no fear of aggravating the condition because ethyl chloride does not mask major lesion or bone damage. If the spraying has no effect, you may have suffered a major ligament tear or tear of the Achilles tendon. These injuries require surgery.

If you suffer an ankle sprain that requires more than one treatment, do the exercises listed below. Be sure to rest several seconds between each exercise. If you become tired or feel pain, stop exercising immediately.

These exercises are to be performed lying down with a large pillow under the knee of the injured leg.

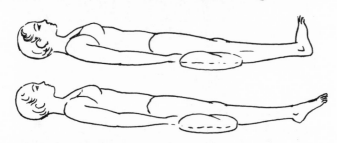

1. Bend and extend the ankle.

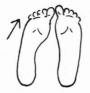 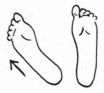

2. Turn the foot in and out.
3. Bend and extend the toes.
When the ankle is strong and comfortable enough to bear weight, add the following exercises.

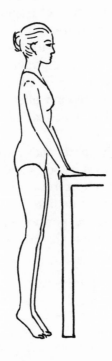

4. Stand on the floor, using a table or chair back for support. Now stand on the toes of both feet and increase weight, as it's tolerated, on the injured ankle.

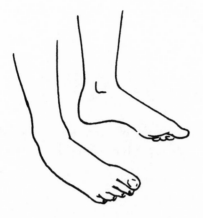

5. Standing, shift weight to the outside of both feet, turn them in, turn them out. If necessary, hold on to a chair or table.

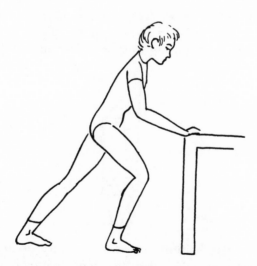

6. Step forward with the injured foot, the knee flexed. Plant the heel firmly on the floor, now bend the knee as far forward as possible without lifting the heel.

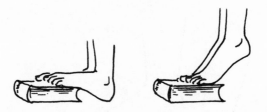

7. Place the forward part of your feet on a book, heels on the floor. Stand on your toes. Now let down, put your heels on the floor.

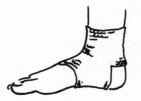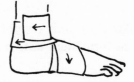

A rubber anklet or an Ace bandage wrapped in a figure eight around the ankle as shown can serve as added protection for a person returning to sports after ankle injury.

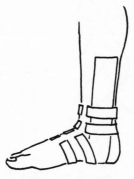

Taping is also helpful, either after injury or to help support an unstable ankle. Run two long two-inch-wide tapes across the instep and up both sides like a stirrup. Then tape shorter strips across as shown. To avoid swelling, do not wrap the entire ankle in tape.

If you suffer from chronically recurring ankle sprain, you should seek medical attention. Sprains can recur when a major tear has been overlooked and not repaired. This is rare, but it does happen. More frequently, incomplete reconditioning after previous injury is the cause of recurring sprains.

10

Rehabilitation After Injury:
The Neck and Back

NECK STRAIN

Most whiplash injuries are muscle strains. As such, they should not be immobilized or placed in collars or traction because this only serves to weaken and stiffen the neck muscles. Cervical collars and rigid neck braces should only be used in cases of mechanical derangement. Some cases of tension headache are caused by tight occipital muscles in the back of the neck. Both neck strain and tension headache can be alleviated with the following relaxation exercises, first performed lying down, then sitting. Use ethyl chloride spray or ice to relieve pain as you move.

1. Lie on your back. Turn your neck to the left, let go, and return to normal. Now turn your neck to the right, let go, and return.

2. Breathe deeply and slowly exhale. Now shrug your shoulders as you inhale, then exhale as you relax your shoulders.

3. Sit on a chair, feet apart on the floor. Let your neck droop, then drop your shoulders and arms, and bend down

between your knees as far as you can go. Return to an upright position and relax.

4. Do exercise 2 sitting.
5. Do exercise 1 sitting.

Repeat exercises in reverse order.

Note that some cases of headache, chronic neck pain, and pain in the upper back may be caused by bite problems. Every examination of chronic pain in these areas should include appraisal of the bite and temperomandibular joint. Most orthodontists are familiar with the problem, which they relieve by correcting the bite and treating the muscles involved.

BACK PAIN

When I began practice in the United States, many of my patients were skiers and track athletes. In fact I treated so many skiers that they called me "Ski Doctor." Then I later worked in the Department of Physical Therapy at Columbia Presbyterian Medical Center, where I joined Dr. Sonja Weber at the hospital's Posture Clinic. There we studied some 400 youngsters who had poor posture.

Our study lasted four years. During that time Dr. Weber and I conducted detailed examinations and tests. One of our first observations showed that the children were quick to assume good posture when examined, but reverted to poor posture when they thought they were not being watched. It occurred to us that poor posture might be the result of muscular inability to move properly. To check this hypothesis we devised a number of tests that would measure the strength and flexibility of the hip, back, and abdominal muscles used to hold the body erect. After constantly comparing results, we finally keyed in on a battery of six tests which are known as the Kraus-Weber Tests. Widely used in physical medicine today, the K-W Tests are shown here. You may want to take them yourself to see if your back is fit.

K-W Test No. 1

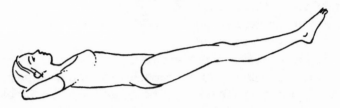

This test is designed to show whether the hip flexors are strong enough. You lie flat on your back with your hands clasped behind your neck and with your legs extended and touching. Keeping your knees straight, raise both feet so that your heels are ten inches above the floor, as shown here. If you can hold this position for ten seconds, you pass this test.

K-W Test No. 2

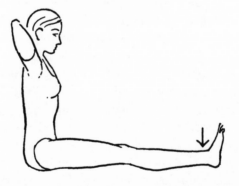

This test shows whether the hip flexors *and* abdominal muscles combined have sufficient strength to handle your body weight. Again lie flat with your hands clasped behind your neck. Have an assistant hold your legs down by grasping the ankles as shown. If you can do one sit-up by rolling up into a sitting position, you pass this test.

K-W Test No. 3

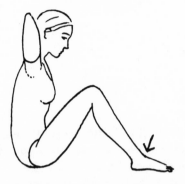

This tests the strength of the abdominal muscles. As before, lie flat on the floor with your hands clasped behind your neck, only this time have your knees flexed as shown. Have your assistant hold down your ankles. You pass if you can roll up into a sitting position.

K-W Test No. 4

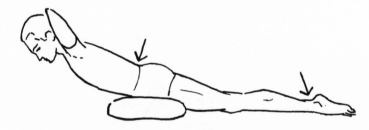

This tests the strength of the back muscles. Turn over on your stomach. Put a large pillow under your abdomen and clasp your hands behind your neck. Have your assistant steady the lower half of your body by placing one hand on the small of your back and the other on your ankles. You pass if you can lift your trunk off the floor and hold it steady for ten seconds.

K-W Test No. 5

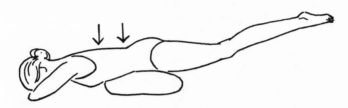

This tests the strength of the low-back muscles. Stay on your stomach and fold your arms under your head with the pillow still beneath your abdomen. Have your assistant steady your back with both hands. You pass if you can raise your legs with the knees straight as shown and hold the position for ten seconds.

K-W Test No. 6

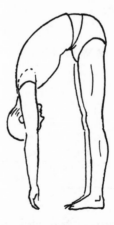

This tests the flexibility of the back muscles and hamstrings. Stand up straight, feet together. Slowly reach down as far as you can without bending the knees. You pass if you can touch the floor. If you fail, it is not because your arms are too short or your legs too long, but because the back and hamstring muscles are shortened and tense.

The K-W Tests permitted us to determine which muscles were weak or inflexible in each child and to understand clinically why certain youngsters had sway backs, round shoulders, or protruding stomachs. We then gave each child a prescribed set of exercises designed to correct the particular deficiency. Those who did not do the exercises reverted to poor posture.

Just as we were concluding our studies in the Posture Clinic, Dr. Barbara Stimson asked us to participate in a special back-pain clinic she had established at Columbia Presbyterian under the direction of Drs. William Darrach and Clay Ray Murray. As part of a team of orthopedic surgeons, neurosurgeons, internists, and psychiatrists, we examined some 3,000 adult patients who had back pain. All patients were X-rayed and given laboratory tests. Dr. Weber and I gave them the K-W Tests, and the majority failed at least one of the six. After reviewing all data, Dr. Sawnie Gaston determined that 83 percent of the patients showed no pathology, such as ruptured discs. Dr. Weber and I prescribed exercises to these muscularly deficient patients, and the results were soon evident. Sixty-five percent of the group were completely without pain, 26 percent had only occasional discomfort, and 9 percent did not respond to treatment. Long-range follow-up of this group revealed that 82 percent had complete recovery and no back pain, 15 percent had occasional discomfort, and 5 percent experienced no relief.

Shortly after our work at Columbia Presbyterian Medical Center, we began giving the K-W Tests to so-called "healthy" children in the general population. We discovered that a high percentage of them failed at least one. In the light of our experience at the back clinic, we felt these youngsters were prime candidates for future back problems.

Back pain was then becoming a widespread complaint throughout the United States, and Dr. Weber and I began to speculate on the reasons why. All sorts of persons in all walks of life, from members of the armed forces to housewives and business executives, suffered from it. Few occupations were spared. We began to wonder if sedentary and stressful living was causing muscles to become weak and tense. In 1947, in an attempt to determine whether or not this was the case, we decided to test two groups of children, one in the United States, the other in Europe. We first administered the K-W Tests to 5,000 U.S. youngsters between the ages of six and sixteen. They had all the medical care that an affluent society could lavish upon them, but they were also growing up in a culture that unconsciously discouraged routine daily exercise through the use of the automobile and the proliferation of television.

We found that most of these supposedly healthy youngsters had weak and tense muscles. Indeed, a majority of them, 57.9 percent to be precise, failed at least one of the K-W Tests. By contrast, 3,000 European youngsters we tested in Switzerland, Austria, and Italy, less mechanized than the United States at the time, did far better. A total of 91.3 percent of these European children passed all the K-W Tests. It is interesting that as these European countries have caught up with the American mechanized standard of living, the rate of failure on the tests now approaches that in the United States. According to Dr. Willi Nagler, now chief of the Department of Physical Medicine and Rehabilitation at Cornell Medical School, the rate of failure by Austrian children almost doubled within a decade as Austria recovered from the war and moved into prosperity replete with automobiles, TV sets, and other appliances.

I wrote widely on the problem. A paper I published in the *New York State Journal of Medicine* was reprinted in a magazine put out by the Amateur Athletic Union. John B. Kelly, who had won three Olympic gold medals for rowing, brought it to the attention of President Dwight Eisenhower. The president held a sports luncheon at the White House, where

I gave a paper on the deplorable physical state of American children. President Eisenhower was shocked. He subsequently established the Council for Youth Fitness, now the President's Council on Physical Fitness and Sports.

DISC MISDIAGNOSIS

Despite all the papers that have poured forth in recent years on the causes of back pain, the condition is often misdiagnosed. A person suffering from weak and deficient back muscles or triggerpoints is told that he or she has a "herniated disc." To avoid surgery, the patient is advised to "live with" the pain and to give up running, tennis, or any "excessive motion." What happens then? The patient is inactive physically, the muscles become weaker and tighter, the triggerpoints (if present) grow worse, and the pain increases in intensity and duration. Minor spurts of physical activity, like picking up a suitcase, turning a doorknob, or even sneezing only inflict more pain on the deteriorating muscles and the sensitive triggerpoints. This downward trend is difficult to reverse. Prompted by the patient's increasing anxieties—fear of surgery, fear of disability, fear of loss of livelihood—more complications develop. In time the patient loses all sense of physical and emotional well-being and becomes resigned to inactivity and constant pain instead of enjoying a life of activity and vigor.

And what happens if this desperate patient finally decides to undergo surgery for a disc problem that does not exist? Postsurgery confinement in a hospital bed only makes the muscles more weak and tense and the triggerpoints still more sensitive. The problem gets worse, and the patient slides into a downward cycle of despair.

Certainly disc problems do occur, and in cases that truly involve a disc, surgery is beneficial. But remember that more than 80 percent of all back pain is caused by muscular deficiency, not by discs. The first thing we do with a back-pain patient is to insist that the patient first be seen by an internist and that X rays be taken. When there is no pathology, we give the patient a thorough neurological examination. If this is negative, we evaluate the patient's muscles for strength, tension, flexibility, and triggerpoints, and we then start on appropriate treatment.

If our conservative treatment does not produce results and pain continues, we refer the patient to a neurologist or a neurosurgeon for further investigation. The neurologist or neurosurgeon then may order an electromyogram, a CAT scan and, if needed, a myelogram. A myelogram is usually not ordered unless disc surgery is contemplated.

Back pain of muscular origin can be relieved with ethyl chloride spray, ice massage, or the application of hot towels. If no triggerpoints are present, you should start doing the exercises given below after you obtain your physician's permission. Except for cases involving mechanical derangement, which is not discussed in this book, I rarely allow patients to wear a back brace because it can weaken support muscles.

I designed these exercises for the YMCA and its Y's Way to a Healthy Back program. So far, more than 150,000 people have finished the program with excellent results. Do the first four exercises the first day. If you feel no discomfort, add a new exercise every other day until you are doing the full program of eighteen exercises. Do each exercise three times and then repeat them in reverse order so that the full program goes 1 through 18, then 17 back to 1.

Exercise 1

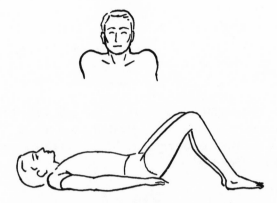

Take a deep breath, then exhale slowly. Now shrug and breathe in. Exhale as you let go of the shrug.

Exercise 2

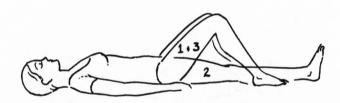

Position yourself comfortably on your back on the floor with both knees bent. Close your eyes. Take a deep breath and exhale slowly. Slide your right leg forward and slide it back. Slide the left leg forward and slide it back. Take another deep breath. Tighten both fists, then let go.

Exercise 3

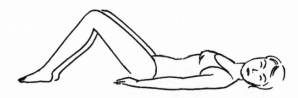

Turn your head all the way to the left, then return it to the normal front and center position, and let go. Turn your head all the way to the right, as far as you can, return to normal position, and relax.

Exercise 4

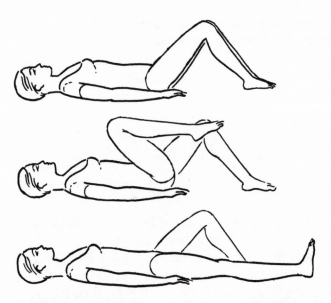

Flex your knees and slowly draw your right knee up as close to your chest as you can comfortably. Return foot to floor, slide the leg forward, and slide it back. Now bring the left leg up to the chest. Return foot to floor, slide the leg forward, and slide it back.

Exercise 5

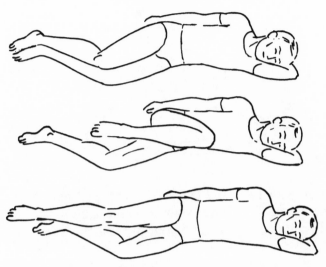

Lie on your left side with your head resting comfortably on your arm. Keep both knees flexed and hips slightly flexed. Slide your right knee as close to your head as is comfortably possible, then slowly extend the leg until it is completely straight. The leg is dead weight; you don't lift your right leg, you slide it on the left leg. Do the exercise three times, then turn to your right side and repeat the exercise with your left leg. Remember, the top leg is dead weight.

Exercise 6

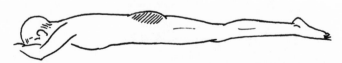

Turn over on your stomach. Let your head rest comfortably on your folded hands and point your toes inward. Now tighten your seat muscles. Hold that position for two seconds, then let go.

Exercise 7: Double Knee Flex

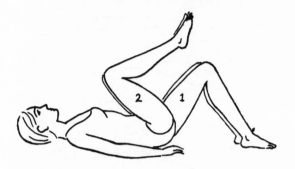

Lie on your back and flex both knees. Pull both knees up to your chest. Then lower your legs gradually to floor in the flexed position. Do not raise your hips off the floor.

Exercise 8: Cat Back

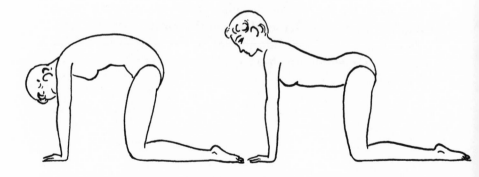

Assume a kneeling position, resting on your hands and knees. Arch your back like a cat and drop your head at the same time. Now reverse the arch by bringing up your head and forming a U with your spine.

Exercise 9: Head Up, Supine

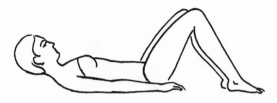

Lie on the floor with knees flexed, hands loose by your sides. Raise your head and shoulders off the floor, bring them down slowly, and relax.

Exercise 10: Pectoral Stretch

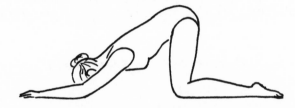

From a kneeling position, place your hands, then your forearms on the floor. Gradually straighten your back, sliding forward on your arms and keeping your back and head straight. This will stretch your pectoral muscles as you move away from your knees. Return to the starting position by walking back up with your arms. Thighs are always perpendicular to the floor.

Exercise 11: Bend Sitting

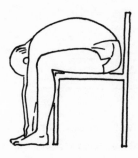

Sit on a chair, feet apart on the floor. Let your neck droop, then drop your shoulders and arms, and bend down between your knees as far as you can. Return to an upright position, straighten up, and relax. Do not force your downward bend.

Exercise 12: Sit-up, Knees Flexed

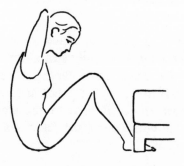

Lie on your back with your hands clasped behind your head, knees flexed. Tuck your feet under a heavy object that won't topple (a chest of drawers, bed or heavy chair, for example). Sit up, then lower yourself slowly to a lying position. You should sit up gradually, first by raising your head, then your shoulders, and then your chest and lower end of

the spine. Do not sit up by holding your trunk stiff and jerking your weight up. If you cannot do this exercise with your
hands behind your neck, try to do it with your hands at your
sides. Later, cross them over your stomach, and still later,
when you are stronger, bring your crossed arms up to your
chest and, finally, behind your neck and head. If you're unable to do this exercise at all, continue with the earlier exercises until you have gained enough strength to manage this
one. Before each sit-up take a deep breath, and exhale as you
curl to a sit-up position.

Exercise 13: Bend Sitting Rotation

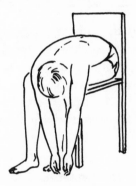

Sit on a chair, bend down, dropping your head and shoulders. Bend down to the left, then gradually straighten up,
rest. Do the exercise again, bending to the right.

Exercise 14: Hamstring Stretch

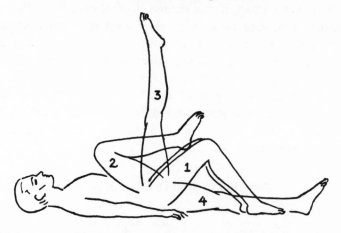

Lie on your back with both knees flexed, arms at sides. Bring your right knee up as close as possible to your chest, extend your right leg, pointing the toes toward the ceiling. Keeping the knee straight, lower your leg to the floor. Then slide the leg back up to the bent position. Do the same for the left leg. Repeat this exercise with your heel instead of toe pointing up.

Exercise 15: Hamstring Stretch

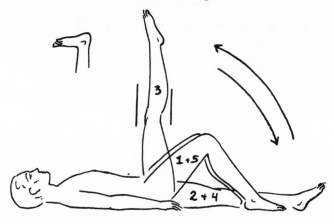

Lie on your back with knees flexed, slide your right leg out, pointing the toes away from your head. Lock the knee and raise your leg as high as you can without bending. Lower the straight leg to floor and slide it to bent position. Do same for the left leg. Repeat this exercise with heel instead of toe pointing up.

Exercise 16: Hamstring Stretch

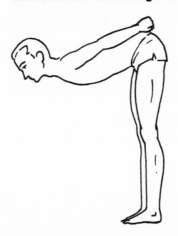

Stand up with heels together and clasp your hands behind your back, keeping your back and neck straight. Bend forward from the hips, gradually lower your trunk, and go down as far as you can, raising your head until you feel stretching in the back of your legs.

Exercise 17: Calf Muscle Stretch

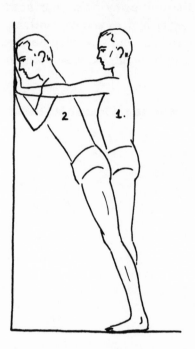

Stand a little bit less than arm's length away from the wall with feet together. Keep hips and back straight and place hands flat on wall. Bending your elbows and using your forearms, slowly allow your straight body to come close to the wall. Then straighten your arms to push your body to the standing position. Always keep your hands in contact with the wall and heels in touch with the floor when leaning into the wall.

Exercise 18: Floor Touch

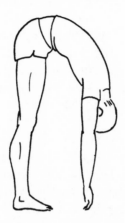

Keep your heels together. Relax by inhaling and exhaling deeply. Drop your neck gradually and let your trunk "hang" loosely from your hips. Drop your shoulders and then your back gradually. Let gravity help you. Do this two or three times. When you're completely relaxed and "hanging from the hips," slowly reach as far down as you can without straining. Relax again, straighten up. Now reverse the order of exercises, going from 17 through 1.

When you are able to do all eighteen exercises satisfactorily, take the K-W Tests again. If you pass all six, and the Minimum Sports Fitness Test in chapter 2, you're fit for sports, but keep your muscles in shape by doing the daily Sports Fitness Exercises in chapter 3.

If you've suffered from back pain for a long time, you may be surprised at how well the eighteen-exercise program will recondition your muscles. On occasion, a back problem may be complicated by another condition, such as endocrine imbalance. Let me cite the case of Mary N., a thirty-year-old professional dancer who came to our clinic six years after she first suffered back pain. The first episode occurred during an evening performance when she had been so rushed that she had no time to warm up. As she bent over while dancing, her low-back muscles suddenly went into spasm. This incident was soon followed by other episodes of pain and spasm. She had tried resistive and stretching exercises, and although they seemed to help, the pain kept returning. In the course of the years she had to cancel several dancing engagements because of pain and spasm, and she was fearful that her career was at an end. When she saw us, she also complained of a pain in her neck.

Examination disclosed that Mary had a triggerpoint in her right suboccipital muscle in the back of her neck and three triggerpoints in her lower back and right hip. She was very tense and complained of constipation, depression, menstrual irregularity, and dry skin. After I treated the triggerpoints, the pain disappeared, and I put her on exercise therapy. I also referred her to an endocrinologist who diagnosed hypothyroidism and started her on thyroid. A month later, Mary returned to our clinic complaining of recurrent pain in her right gluteal muscle. I found a triggerpoint that had previously been obscured, injected it, and relieved the discomfort. That was ten years ago. Mary resumed her career. A few years ago she began teaching dance. She has had no pain or back problem since.

11

Rehabilitation After Fracture

What do you do in the event you suffer a fracture? The first thing you should do is to see a physician as soon as possible. Bone fragments may have to be brought into proper alignment. A fracture may require immobilization or surgery. After treatment or surgery, you can then begin to exercise as soon as your physician permits by doing the appropriate exercises described previously for strains and sprains. If you broke your wrist, do the wrist exercises. If you broke your leg, do the leg exercises, and so on.

FRACTURES WITHOUT DISPLACEMENT

A number of fractures—fractures without displacement of bone—can be treated with immediate mobilization. Some years ago I worked with Dr. Jesse Mahoney, the chief of fracture surgery at Bellevue Hospital in New York, and we found that a number of fractures often lent themselves to immediate mobilization. They are:

impacted fractures of the head of the humerus, the bone running from the shoulder joint to the elbow
fractures of the plateau or upper end of the tibia, the shin bone

fractures of the metatarsals, the long bones of the foot

fractures of the calcaneus, the heel bone

fractures of the lateral malleolus of the ankle without displacement

fractures of the pubic ramus of the pelvis

fractures of the vertebrae if no pedicles are involved

fractures of the transverse process of vertebrae and other fractures of the vertebrae that did not endanger the spinal cord

fractures of the metacarpal bones, the long bones of the hand

fractures of the phalanges, the finger bones

Don't infer from reading this that you can run out and play right after you break a bone, although as you'll see, I had a patient who did. But what you can do in most instances is to get a head start on recovery by exercising the muscles right away. Let me cite the case history of Peter E., a vigorous man in his mid-thirties and a first-rate downhill skier. Several years ago he fell and hurt his upper right arm while racing. He immediately saw an orthopedist who found that Peter had an impacted fracture of the head of the humerus. After swathing the arm in bandages and putting it in a sling, the orthopedist advised Peter to see us. Six days after the accident, Peter came in for his first treatment. We removed the bandages, sprayed the shoulder and arm with ethyl chloride, and had Peter do gentle exercises for the arm and shoulder muscles. He returned twice that week for further treatment, and when we saw him the next week, we asked how he felt.

"Great!" he exclaimed. "There's still a slight ache in the shoulder, but it's easy for me to ski even with my arm in the sling."

"Hold on," I said. "You have an impacted fracture, and you're a fool to ski. No more skiing until I say so."

After a few weeks, the fracture had healed. He had full

range and power in his arm and shoulder and no pain whatever. He then returned to skiing, and he has had no problem
since.

Here are a couple of other cases of fractures without displacement. Several years ago, I was looking forward to a
mountain-climbing vacation in Italy with my old friend
Gino Solda, a celebrated resistance fighter in World War II
and one of the great mountaineers in the world. When I
arrived in Gino's village, I was disappointed to find him in
bed with his right foot encased in plaster. He had just broken
two short bones in his foot, and his doctor had put him
in plaster and confined him to bed. I looked at the X rays,
removed the plaster, and had Gino exercise the leg. Two
days later, he walked to the foot of a cliff and watched me
climb, and a week later we were climbing the Dolomites
together.

The son of a very close friend fell while skiing and broke
the pubic ramus of the pelvis. He was taken to the local
hospital and put in a hammock. This consisted of a firm cloth
suspended at both ends, with the patient's pelvis resting in
it elevated from the bed. The patient's father asked me to
examine him because the son was extremely uncomfortable
and unable to perform bodily functions. He was scheduled
to spend six weeks in the hammock. In addition to the discomfort, he was going to lose a semester in college. I was
courteously received by the local surgeon, and immediately
removed the young man from the hammock. Using ethyl
chloride spray to relieve pain, I started the patient on movement. He was able to sit up, pass urine, and move his bowels.
The next day he came to New York by ambulance, and after
further treatment he was back in college on crutches in a
week. I must give special credit to that local surgeon. Soon
afterwards an older woman suffered the same fracture, but
this time instead of using the hammock, he treated her the
same way I had treated my friend's son. Nowadays, few
hospitals use a hammock for fracture of the pelvis, but en-

forced bed rest is still prevalent, and that is not a good practice.

FATIGUE OR STRESS FRACTURES

Fatigue or stress fractures occur in the short and long bones of the foot, tibia, fibula, and sometimes the femur. They are caused by overstrain, such as by doing a lot of running, especially downhill, or marching with a heavy pack. Troops in training sometimes suffer them. It takes two or three weeks for fatigue fractures to show up on an X ray, but a bone scan will detect them immediately. Fatigue fractures of the tibia can often be distinguished from shin splints by noting the source of tenderness or pain. With shin splints the muscles are tender to the touch, while with fatigue fractures the bone is tender. Fatigue fractures usually take six to eight weeks to heal. The patient should use crutches until able to walk without pain or limping. Meanwhile, the appropriate foot and/or leg exercises should be done.

FRACTURED RIB

Aside from relieving muscle spasm with ethyl chloride spray and gentle limbering exercises, we leave a broken rib or ribs alone. We do not tape. We give the patient an analgesic and a sleeping pill at night, but no medication during the day. Later, we have the patient do the back exercises described in chapter 10 because they condition all the key muscle groups that could be affected by inactivity.

EXERCISING AFTER SURGERY

If surgery is required for a fracture, rehabilitation exercises should be started as soon as possible afterwards with the surgeon's approval. This may be immediately after plaster has been applied. My great teacher, Dr. William Darrach, the chief of fracture surgery at Columbia Presbyterian Medical Center, always said, "The best way to treat a fracture is to wish the bones in place. Keep the bones there with a wish and start exercises at once." His associate, Dr. Clay Ray Murray, concurred. As soon as the fracture was reduced and stabilized in proper position, we began exercising the affected muscles so they could regain full strength and flexibility. Early mobilization speeds up healing.

If you wonder how you can exercise while encased in plaster, let me give you an example. Let's say that you've undergone surgery for a severe ankle fracture. Following surgery, your leg is immobilized in plaster from the foot to above the knee. As soon as the plaster has been applied and you're in bed, you can begin exercising. There is no way you can do ankle exercises per se, but you can bend and extend your toes frequently, do leg raises, and tighten your quadriceps. When the plaster is cut down below the knee, you can start doing the knee exercises shown in chapter 9. Keep in mind that your whole leg has been immobilized, not just the ankle, and that all the leg muscles have to be brought back to full strength and flexibility. After a while you may be permitted to walk in the plaster, provided you have full knee extension. The plaster will support your weight. However, once the plaster is removed, avoid unaided walking until you can do so without limping and without pain. Start doing the ankle exercises. Your ankle and leg muscles must be restored to full strength and flexibility before you walk without crutches. I cannot repeat this point enough. Always remember that even when a fracture is healed, the muscles in the affected part are not as strong and as flexible as they were before the fracture. This is especially important to keep in mind about fractures of the lower extremities because they bear your body weight.

Let's say that you weigh 160 pounds, and you're now told that your ankle fracture has healed. If you're also informed that you can now recondition yourself by walking a quarter of a mile on your own the first day, a half mile the second day, and so on, don't you do it unless the leg muscles are strong enough and flexible enough to bear your own body weight fully without pain. If you weigh 160 pounds, you should have a 160-pound leg, that is, a leg capable of supporting your weight. You can check the strength of your leg by doing the bathroom-scale test on page 105.You may find that you have only an 80-pound leg. You must do more leg exercises until the leg can support your weight on the scale. What would happen if you began walking unassisted with an 80-pound leg? You'd be asking it to do a 160-pound job, and it would soon show the strain. The first day out, you'd have a little pain in the leg after walking. The next day, the leg would have more pain. The pain comes from weak and tight muscles. If you continued to walk, you would have constant pain in the leg, even when at rest. Soon you would begin to walk with the leg as though it were a stilt. This would stiffen the muscles even more, and permanent disability could result.

I well remember the sad case of Jan S., who was twenty-five when she came to see us. She had been a good downhill and cross-country skier until she suffered a fractured left femur, tibia, and pelvis in an automobile accident a year and a half before. Jan's fractures were beautifully taken care of in surgery, and she then went through eight months of immobilization in plaster while they healed. During this time, Jan did no exercises at all, but when she was discharged from the hospital, she was told she could walk as much as she wished.

Jan did, and she was soon suffering pain in her left leg. A

hardy young woman, she continued to walk, thinking she could recondition her leg by "walking it out." After all, she was young, and she had led an active life physically. In time her leg stiffened so much it resembled a bent stick. It was then that she came to see us.

Examination revealed that Jan's ankle and knee were completely frozen. To put it bluntly, she had a useless leg. We started Jan on exercise therapy.

It took us a full year to restore Jan's leg muscles to reasonable strength and flexibility and to straighten out the knee so that she had complete movement without pain. She also recovered full range of the upper part of her ankle, but not of the lower part, the subtalar joint. The damage to the subtalar joint was permanent. She never will be able to turn her foot in or move her ankle from side to side. She can't dance, she can't play tennis, and she can't ski downhill because she can't edge with her ankle. She does manage to do some cross-country skiing, but even here she is handicapped. Her active life has been needlessly cut short because she walked before her leg could bear her body weight.

12

A Caution
for the Young and Old

Very young children, those from the age of three to six, can be started on sports, but they should not be pushed beyond their abilities. Certainly youngsters of this age should be given the opportunity to exercise and use their bodies instead of storing up tension by watching television.

As youngsters grow, they often want to take part in competitive sports. There is a risk here, but competitive sports are permissible if not done to excess. It is better to take potential injuries in stride than to prevent a youngster from participating in healthful physical activity. Care must be taken, however. The growth areas of the bones are especially sensitive to injury and should be protected.

If you are elderly, don't stop your sporting endeavors even though your abilities have decreased. Remaining physically and mentally active is the best antidote to premature aging.

As you get older, your warm-up has to be more thorough, and it will take more time. This is because the jelling time of your muscles decreases with age. They jell much more quickly than the muscles of a younger person. You can see this if you and your grandchild sit down for ten or fifteen minutes. Your grandchild will pop out of the chair easily while you will feel a certain stiffness.

Bear in mind that your abilities have become limited, and if you try to keep up with the sporting goals of the past and push yourself to the limit, you will be functioning at your maximum but not at your optimum. You're competing with your own younger age, and you can't win that race. It also exposes you to injury. Don't start a new sport unless you're willing to accept the increased risk of injury.

The fact that you're losing some of your strength and flexibility doesn't mean that you should no longer play sports but that you should try for less ambitious goals. Don't fret about this. Nature is kind to you. Even though you are unable to accomplish as much as in the past, you can still get the same sense of exhilaration, the same "high," on a lower level that you experienced in the extreme in your younger days of triumph. Don't let the knowledge that what you do now does not compare favorably with what you did previously interfere with your joy in sports.

If you have been bedridden for a relatively short time or suffered an injury that requires immobilization, exercise the injured parts of your body as best you can. If bedridden, you should have periods of exercise compatible with your medical problem. More often than not you will be able to do some of the exercises prescribed for back pain in chapter 10, and be sure to do breathing exercises to keep your lungs well ventilated.

Index